EAT LIKE AN ATHLETE

Published in 2019 by Hardie Grant Books,
an imprint of Hardie Grant Publishing

Hardie Grant Books (Melbourne)
Building 1, 658 Church Street
Richmond, Victoria 3121

Hardie Grant Books (London)
5th & 6th Floors
52–54 Southwark Street
London SE1 1UN

hardiegrantbooks.com

All rights reserved. No part of this publication may be reproduced, stored in a retrieval system or transmitted in any form by any means, electronic, mechanical, photocopying, recording or otherwise, without the prior written permission of the publishers and copyright holders.

The moral rights of the author have been asserted.

Copyright text © Simone Austin 2019

A catalogue record for this book is available from the National Library of Australia

Eat Like An Athlete

ISBN 978 1 74379 468 5

10 9 8 7 6 5 4 3 2 1

Cover design by Sinéad Murphy

Text design by Sinéad Murphy

Typeset in 10/14 pt FreightText Pro by Sinéad Murphy

Cover image courtesy of Stocksy; back cover images courtesy of FatFree Agency, Unsplash, Shutterstock

Printed by McPherson's Printing Group, Maryborough, Victoria

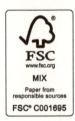

The paper this book is printed on is certified against the Forest Stewardship Council® Standards. FSC® promotes environmentally responsible, socially beneficial and economically viable management of the world's forests.

About the Author

Simone Austin is an advanced sports dietitian and an accredited practising dietitian. Simone is passionate about making nutritious food choices the easy choices, to help people maximise their health and performance.

Simone has a proven track record as an advanced sports dietitian, having worked in elite sport with a range of successful teams and individuals. She has been working at Hawthorn Football Club for ten years, during which time the club won three AFL premierships. She helped the Australian Men's Cricket team to two World Cups and an Ashes victory, and the Melbourne Storm to a premiership win. In her long career, Simone has also worked with Melbourne City soccer club (Melbourne Heart at the time) and the Melbourne Rebels Rugby Union team, as well as junior AFL teams and individual athletes.

Simone has provided nutrition advice to many of Australia's elite professional athletes, including Leisel Jones, Ricky Ponting, Glenn McGrath, Brad Johnson, Luke Hodge, Cyril Rioli, Cooper Cronk and Billy Slater. Simone loves addressing grassroots sporting clubs and inspiring junior athletes to eat well in order to maximise their own sporting performance and health, just like their sporting idols.

Simone is President of Sports Dietitians Australia and a media spokesperson for the Dietitians Association of Australia. Her love of food motivates her to spread practical, accurate nutrition advice, and her engaging, compassionate nature inspires people to 'eat like an athlete' and discover how they can use food to maximise performance in all areas of life.

You can read more about Simone, her nutrition tips and stories on her website www.simoneaustin.com, and follow her for daily tips on Instagram (@simone_austin), on Facebook (Simone Austin Dietitian) or on Twitter (@simonejaustin).

SIMONE AUSTIN ADVANCED SPORTS DIETITIAN

EAT LIKE AN ATHLETE

BOOST YOUR PERFORMANCE AND ENERGY THROUGH NUTRITION

Hardie Grant

BOOKS

Table of Contents

PREFACE		1
INTRODUCTION		7
SECTION 1	**FOOD AND YOUR BODY**	10
Chapter 1	The First Steps to Eating Like an Athlete	11
Chapter 2	The Carbohydrate Guide	27
Chapter 3	Protein	49
Chapter 4	Fat: The Good, the Bad and the Ugly	57
Chapter 5	Fluid and Hydration	63
Chapter 6	Is Alcohol Allowed?	77
Chapter 7	Salt	83
Chapter 8	The Immune System	87
Chapter 9	Maximising Your Gut's Performance	93
Chapter 10	Superfoods	115

SECTION 2	EATING FOR PERFORMANCE AND RECOVERY	122
Chapter 11	What Should I Eat Before Exercise?	123
Chapter 12	What to Eat on Game Day	129
Chapter 13	Strategies for a Speedy Recovery	139
Chapter 14	Do Nutrition Needs Change with Age?	151

SECTION 3	STRATEGIES FOR HEALTHY EATING	166
Chapter 15	Making Lifestyle Changes	167
Chapter 16	Making Life Easier in the Kitchen	187
Chapter 17	Quick Meal Ideas	201
Chapter 18	How to Successfully Eat Out	215
Chapter 19	Eating at Celebrations	223
Chapter 20	Healthy Eating While Travelling	233

CONCLUSION	240

Preface

What could be better, or easier, than good, simple food, and the pleasure of sharing it with others? It should be straightforward, but we are constantly receiving contradictory messages about healthy eating, and being exposed to new fad diets. As a result, nutrition has become confusing, and doing the right thing seems impossibly hard. So where do you begin?

Healthy eating doesn't have to be complicated, hard work or expensive. It means fuelling your body, rather than depriving it, and examining your food intake and health with a positive outlook. Athletes use nutrition as a tool to maximise peak performance, and you can too.

Food can be enjoyable. It can also maximise your energy levels, health and performance. Find out how you can give your body the optimal nourishment it requires.

It doesn't matter what your activity level is – eating like an athlete will help you perform at your best. Whether you want to improve your time in a triathlon or marathon (or compete in your first), boost your performance at the gym, feed an active child, or want to be able to cycle or hike in your retirement, *Eat Like An Athlete* is for you. Make the most of your physical activity by complementing it with optimal nutrition, which is often the missing part of the performance equation.

This book will provide key nutritional information and offer practical suggestions to help you establish a healthy diet that meets your physical activity requirements. It will answer the questions that I am often asked, such as: Should I eat before exercise? What should I eat before exercise and competition? How much protein do I need for muscle gain and/or maintenance? What about carbohydrates? What are good breakfast choices to get me through the day, and how do I avoid the 3 pm energy slump? How much fluid do I need?

I will share stories about what has worked, and why, and pass on knowledge gained from my extensive experience working with elite athletes, sports teams and amateur sports enthusiasts, translating the science into everyday practice. This book is designed to be a resource for everyone who is interested in understanding and improving their nutrition and performance.

HOW TO USE THIS BOOK

Eat Like An Athlete is divided into three sections:

- » Section 1 provides technical nutritional information (pages 10–120).
- » Section 2 discusses specific topics relating to competing/performing as an athlete (pages 122–164).
- » Section 3 offers tips on how to put the knowledge from sections 1 and 2 into practice (pages 166–239).

You can read the book from cover to cover or flip to the topic that most interests you. You may wish to revisit a section when your needs change. You can also look for tips on specific topics, such as what to do when travelling (chapter 20, starting on page 233), ideas for healthy dinners (page 212) or what to eat before training (chapter 12, starting on page 123).

The notes section included at the back of the book provides room to write down your goals and strategies, and to jot down conversations you might want to have with key people who influence your diet and health.

With the practical information and achievable tips provided in *Eat Like An Athlete*, you and your family will be able to develop healthy eating habits to live well.

A BIT ABOUT ME

Some of my friends refer to me as a 'pocket rocket', others call me 'The Eveready Bunny'. When I worked at the Australian Men's Cricket team my nickname was 'Mighty Mouse'. People used to comment that they'd seen me running to school pick-up – I thought I was walking! As you may have gathered, I tend to do things quickly, and have a lot of energy.

Being around people energises me. I love seeing the way people beam when you pay them a compliment, or when you carry out a random act of kindness. It makes them feel good, and that makes me feel good, too. For me, love and kindness, together with nutritious food and being active, are the fundamentals of good health.

I tend to eat healthy foods out of desire – I love their taste and the way they make me feel. However, I also enjoy a sweet treat most days, and often read the dessert menu before the main.

Many people assume a dietitian wouldn't want a piece of cake or some chocolate. Some years ago I was filming a short nutrition segment with a chef who, I had been told, was not fond of dietitians. As I arrived, he'd just finished baking a delicious cake. He cut me a generous slice, added a dollop of cream and handed it to me. I was delighted, and dug straight in. He looked shocked. If it was intended as a test, I passed with flying colours, and it was smooth sailing working with him from then on. Moral of the story: we can all enjoy balance, even when striving for an elite nutritional intake, and food is more than the nutrients it provides.

WHEN DID I BECOME INTERESTED IN HEALTH?

One day, in Year 10, I was flicking through the university prospectus books and came across the page about being a dietitian. The profession seemed to incorporate my interests beautifully. I loved food, cooking, sport and being healthy. In my final years of high school, I competed in short-course triathlons and played water polo. Being active was in my blood; my dad played and coached cricket and Aussie Rules football. My parents had also instilled in me good eating habits (and I try to pass these on to my own children). Sports dietetics seemed like the perfect fit.

I completed a Bachelor of Science at Monash University in 1991, and a Masters in Nutrition and Dietetics at Deakin University in 1993. In the final year of my masters, I was able to pick my last student placement, so I approached guru sports dietitian Karen Inge. During the week-long placement I was astounded by the range of work that this field could offer. Sports nutrition had a positive focus, aiming to help athletes maximise performance and be at their best. Karen, along with Lorna Garden (who mentored me), is a leader in our profession, and both women helped introduce sports nutrition at an elite level.

Karen suggested I apply for the position of sports dietitian at the Western Bulldogs AFL team. I was twenty-four years old. My journey in nutrition had begun, and I have been working with elite sports teams ever since. It seems like only yesterday that I was working with the Australian Men's Cricket team, discussing nutrition strategies, while my six-week-old daughter was being nursed by the likes of Steve Waugh, Andrew Symonds and Brett Lee. She is now halfway through high school and helps me collect sweat samples from the Hawthorn players: 'Mum, they smell, and it's not good!'

As well as working with elite sporting groups and individuals, I also keep up my professional development to maintain my advanced sports dietitian and accredited practising dietitian credentials. I volunteer as president at Sports Dietitians Australia, and as a media spokesperson for the Dietitians Association of Australia.

As well as constantly educating myself with the latest research, I also learn from all the clients, health professionals and people I have worked with over the years. This has given me a wealth of knowledge that I would like to share with you now.

MY PHILOSOPHY ON HEALTH

Having a healthy diet doesn't mean you have to spend more, buy 'special' foods, follow a complicated regime or miss out on the foods you enjoy. Eating for health (and like an athlete) can be enjoyable, tasty, fun, energising, practical, convenient, and economically sustainable.

There is more to the equation of health than nutrition. For me, sleeping regular hours is key to sustaining energy levels. My children think I'm too strict about bedtimes, but I know how important sleep is for the body's restoration.

Nowadays, I work being active into my day, more than attending set classes and water polo matches. I find opportunities to be active, such as walking to the train station, the local shops or work, washing my car, gardening, housework and walk-and-talk catch-ups with friends. My household chores are like a gym workout at home without needing a membership. I encourage my children to walk anywhere that is within 1 kilometre. All of this adds up, at no cost or hassle. If you enjoy group sessions like I do (particularly for yoga), fantastic, go for it. Do whatever works for you!

To be sustainable, looking after your health needs to be as simple, enjoyable and practical as possible. Having a goal such as a fun run/walk, cycle event or hike to work towards can be a great motivator to 'eat like an athlete'.

Introduction

WHAT IS HEALTHY EATING?

Healthy eating does not mean dieting. Healthy eating means making food and eating choices that will enable you to live a full and healthy life. It is about establishing good patterns of eating that provide the nutrients you need, make you feel good and that enable you to enjoy food long-term, not making extreme, temporary changes.

Contrary to popular opinion, the nutritional basis of healthy eating is much the same today as it was decades ago. The key messages haven't changed: eat plenty of vegetables, fruits, whole grains, lean meats, fish, nuts, meat alternatives, legumes and dairy. Eat healthy mono- and polyunsaturated fats, less sugar and salt, and fewer highly processed foods, and drink plenty of water. It might sound boring, but if you're doing this, you're on the right track. The technical part is individualising it to you and your needs, including your tastes, activity levels and any medical conditions.

Somewhere along the way, this simple message has became complicated – too much noise has got in the way. There is money to be made in creating confusion, creating new, 'healthier' versions of highly processed foods, and promoting new fad diets. Healthy eating seems to have become overly complicated, but it doesn't need to be.

When my ex-husband was growing up, his grandmother, a Maltese immigrant, would telephone his mother each day and ask, 'Have your children had their egg, banana, orange and milk today?' That was forty-five years ago. Including each of these things in our daily food intake would be an excellent start to good health today!

I see food as a tool to maximise health and performance, regardless of what you are doing in life. The World Health Organization defines health as 'a state of complete physical, mental and social well-being and not merely the absence of disease or infirmity'.

The food we eat is one component that contributes to health. Food's influence on health should be measured by many factors, not just body weight. Blood pressure, blood sugar, blood cholesterol and triglycerides, vitamin and mineral levels, markers of inflammation, bowel health, bone density and energy levels are all key markers of health, and are all influenced by food. Restrictive dieting is not healthy for either the mind or the body.

Healthy eating requires thinking about what you are eating, and spending a little time planning. It is about choosing nutritious foods to fuel your body. Getting in tune with your body's cues, such as hunger, fullness and thirst, can help you develop confidence in eating to your body's needs, rather than by rules or external signals. Importantly, it should also involve eating a wide variety of delicious foods from many food groups, including your favourites. A healthy diet should nourish both your mind and your body.

SECTION 1

FOOD AND YOUR BODY

CHAPTER 1
The First Steps to Eating Like an Athlete

STEP 1. MONITORING, NOT DIETING

Athletes are often asked to track everything, from sleep quality, heart rate and mood to food and fluid intake. They are assessed on how fast they can run, how much weight they can lift – the list goes on. Many athletes like these numbers, and thrive on the feedback. The data can be very useful in adjusting training, competition strategy and lifestyle to ultimately improve performance.

But do we really need to track our food intake that closely, follow prescriptive diets and count kilojoules? I don't believe we do, even as elite athletes. I never 'write diets' for anyone. Instead, I offer guidance by suggesting food choices and educating about composition of certain foods. This enables the athlete to select foods based on sports nutrition principles while still having a choice about what, when and how much they want to eat. A prescriptive diet doesn't allow for adaptation based on what food is available, how the athlete is feeling, changes to training or if injury or illness occurs.

Monitoring, rather than dieting, involves learning about your own body and its needs and desires, along with sports nutrition principles. This gives you the skills and confidence to make your own decisions about your food intake. A sports dietitian helps guide the ship, steering it back on track if it goes off course or needs to change direction.

There are times where nutrients need to be calculated. For example, you might need to add up your protein intake to ensure you are meeting your needs, or checking your carbohydrate intake before an endurance event to ensure you don't run out of fuel. But overall, eating like an athlete means being aware of what you're eating, rather than being overly prescriptive about it.

STEP 2. EATING WITH AWARENESS

Too often I see athletes eat so-called 'perfect diets' for a certain period of time and then, finding it restrictive, antisocial and miserable, throw it all in and just 'eat whatever'. They return to the 'perfect diet' at a later date, and so the cycle continues. Understanding your own cues so you can eat without guilt is a much healthier way to achieve your goals. Try asking yourself the following questions to guide you in what to eat, how much and when:

- » What are my energy levels like?
- » How much fuel will I need for the upcoming session?
- » What do I feel best eating after a match? (Nutrition needs can be met with a broad range of different foods.)
- » How do I feel when I eat a certain food before I train?
- » What do I like to eat?
- » What is practical?
- » What is affordable?

Understanding what you are eating and drinking and how it affects your body is very important. However, there can be a point at which this becomes obsessive and develops into disordered eating, or an eating disorder. We eat and drink for basic survival, but in today's society, food is much more than this. Eating is one of the many enjoyments of life, but with the pressures of body composition and body image, particularly for athletes, we can sometimes become slaves to the dieting world, living a life of restriction and obsession.

There are some strategies we can look at in order to maintain balance, meet goals and find pleasure in eating. Our busy lives mean we often find ourselves eating automatically, paying little attention to what we are eating, or how much. We lose sight of the importance of nourishing our body, and of the pleasure of eating. One commonly discussed strategy is 'mindful eating'. This concept stems from the idea of 'mindfulness', which means paying attention, non-judgementally, to what we are doing. Mindfulness looks at internal and external cues and your mental, physical and emotional state, and focuses on freeing yourself of reactive, habitual behaviours.

Eating with awareness means eating with all of our senses engaged. We first eat with our eyes – I love the saying 'Feast your eyes on this!' Our eyes notice colours and textures, and recognise familiar foods. Then we use our sense of smell, (hopefully) enjoying the fragrance of the food. Hearing also comes into eating – how good is the crunch of a fresh apple? We also use our sense of touch, feeling the texture of the food, possibly with our hands and of course with our mouth and tongue. Then we taste the flavours as we're chewing.

Take some time to consider these questions:

- » What do you do when you're eating? Do you watch television or look at your phone? Do you eat while driving?
- » Are you hungry before you eat? How hungry?
- » Do you eat quickly, finishing the food before you have even had a chance to taste it properly?

When we eat too quickly we often overeat. Because we haven't finished psychologically enjoying the food, we continue, putting more on our plate and often eating past the point of comfort. It takes time for the stomach to tell the brain it has had enough. By eating more slowly, you are more likely to register this message before it is too late.

I find as a parent of young children, it's easy to develop the habit of rushing, because you need to attend to them. A few years ago my daughter, Rebecca, exclaimed 'Mum! You don't have to inhale your food!' That was the wake-up call I needed to slow down. I still need to remind myself to eat slowly, and to focus on what I am eating, not on what I need to do next. I find if I haven't taken the time to enjoy my meal at the end of the evening, I look for food later to 'relax' with. It has nothing to do with being hungry, and can easily lead to overeating.

If you eat while watching television, looking at your phone or with other distractions, your eating will be somewhat robotic. Before you know it, you'll have finished the food without even tasting or enjoying it – and you'll probably find yourself wanting more.

My house has a long hallway. I've noticed that if I prepare myself a post-dinner snack and start eating it in the kitchen, by the time I've walked down the hall to the lounge, it's finished. And because I didn't concentrate on enjoying it, I want more. But if I wait until I'm sitting, concentrate on what I'm eating and relish it, one serve is generally sufficient.

I find that these strategies are particularly important when working with athletes who have large appetites and need to keep lean, such as AFL footballers, Rugby League players and triathletes. Using strategies to eat mindfully can help avoid the feeling of food deprivation, because it means you are enjoying the food and the whole eating experience.

Trust your body to tell you when you are hungry and when you are not. Be patient with yourself – it may take some practice to recognise the signals. Some days you're likely to be hungrier than others, so vary the serving size accordingly, rather than eating the same amount out of habit. Think about hunger as a signal to eat. When you're not hungry, consider whether you really need to eat. Despite what you may have been told when you were young, you don't have to clean your plate – it's okay to leave some.

HUNGER VS. FULLNESS SCALE

A hunger vs. fullness scale is a ranking system used to help you assess how much food you can eat while still feeling comfortable. Many athletes I work with find this scale helpful, and it may be helpful for you too.

» Starving is 1.
» Neutral is 5.
» Too full is 10.

You are comfortably full at around 7–8. Not hungry, not full, just comfortable. If you are unsure whether you are still hungry, wait a while. Drink some water, and maybe go for a walk. You can always get some more food later, when you feel hungry again. Being hungry isn't the same as not being completely full.

Use this scale to rate yourself before and after eating. This can help you decide whether you are eating because you are hungry, or simply for the pleasure of eating. Sometimes we eat purely for pleasure, and that's okay. Being aware that we're doing this can help prevent it from happening too often.

Identifying when you are most hungry during the day also helps with preparation. This information means you can make sure you have suitable meals or snacks ready around those times. Aim to keep yourself between 3 and 7 on the hunger vs. fullness scale. Being too hungry can lead to the release of stress hormones, resulting in a bad mood. This is a natural protective response by the body – it doesn't want to starve.

This is another reason why prescriptive diets tend not to work. When all foods are allowed and nothing is forbidden, this can actually cause you to desire nutritious foods more, and to eat smaller volumes of others. When we deny ourselves certain foods, it's easy to fall into the trap of overeating when we do have those foods, because it can feel like a sort of 'last supper'. Knowing you can eat your favourite food again another time makes it easier to manage how much you eat. Focus on how you feel when you eat mostly nutritious foods, and eat only until you're comfortable.

What are your triggers for mindless eating? Boredom? Being tired? Feeling emotional? Or is it simply habit? Try to develop strategies to help modify your habitual behaviour, such as:

- sitting in a different chair while watching television
- having a glass of water ready
- going for a walk
- buying plenty of healthy food options you would like to eat
- using the hunger vs. fullness scale.

Finding what works for you is the key.

I regularly talk with athletes about eating until they are comfortable, rather than full. Young boys who have had teenage growth spurts requiring lots of food to fuel their growth get used to eating those volumes. When the growth spurt stops, it can be tricky to register that a smaller volume of food is then required. Identifying the difference between eating until comfortable and eating until full is something they all benefit from.

I worked with the Australian Men's Cricket team from 2002 until 2008. One day we were having lunch at the MCG during a Boxing Day test. Andrew Symonds looked at my plate and said, jokingly, 'Is that going to make you 7/10 full?' It was a good reminder for me – overwhelmed by the lovely buffet lunch, I had some of everything on my plate. Of course, I may have just been very hungry that day. Your needs and desires will change each day.

Paying attention to what we eat and why can help us regain some of the pleasure of eating, and decrease the pressure around food. It can take some practice, but before long you'll find it makes an enormous difference to the way you feel. Here are a few tips to get you started.

TIPS FOR EATING WITH AWARENESS

Eating with awareness is a topic that could easily fill a whole book on its own. Here are just a few strategies to start you off:

- Understand your body's natural signals for hunger, comfort and fullness.
- Recognise that, as an athlete, there are times you might need to eat even though you're not hungry (such as recovery time, when you are exhausted and have no appetite, but need to refuel), or when you might need to eat less than you desire (such as when you need to make weight for a weight category sport).
- Develop your own patterns of eating, and remember that these are individual – don't compare yourself to others.
- Choose somewhere to eat where you won't be distracted or tempted to multitask, rather than eating while working away at your desk.
- Try removing distractions: switch off the phone, television and computer, or move away from them, and listen to what your body is telling you. (Are you still hungry? Full? Are you enjoying the food?) Use the fullness vs. hunger scale.
- Before you start eating, take a moment to break the 'rush mode'. Take a few deep breaths to calm yourself, and look at your food. Smell it, and think about what you are about to eat. Concentrate on what's on your plate. The Japanese have a saying that roughly translates to: 'Thank you for the meal. Let's eat.' This stopping and pausing before you dig in helps you move your focus to mindful eating. It acts a bit like a circuit-breaker, shifting you out of the rush of what you were doing before.

> - Taste that first mouthful and really pay attention to the flavours and textures.
> - If you find that you rush your food, and eat until you're overfull, pace yourself with someone who eats slower than you. It can be easy to overeat if you're starving, particularly after exercise.
> - Food is more than just nutrients – slow down and enjoy the occasion. Take it as an opportunity to collect yourself, show gratitude for the meal, and enjoy the surroundings or company you have – they can be part of both the enjoyment and the health benefits.

WHAT ARE YOU ACTUALLY EATING AND DRINKING?

Without becoming obsessive about it, it's worth taking stock of whether you regularly eat as well as you think you do. Nutrition can be balanced over days or weeks, rather than every day or every meal. Are you getting the basic things you need?

- How many servings of vegetables would you have per day, including on weekends?
- Are you eating two servings of fruit a day?
- Are you choosing wholegrain breads and cereals most of the time?
- Do you spread your protein intake out over the day?
- Are you getting enough minerals, such as iron and calcium?
- How often do you eat out?
- How often do you have alcohol?
- How much do you pour for an alcoholic drink? A standard drink of wine is 100 ml, whereas the glasses poured at a restaurant are usually 150 ml.
- Do you have soft drink or other sugary drinks? Look at the supermarket aisles: how much is taken up by soft drink? There are whole aisles of it, so someone must be drinking it!

Look at your dinnerware. Research has shown that eating from larger plates or bowls more likely results in larger portions, as we fill the plate/bowl/glass without thinking about the amount we're putting into it. Downsizing to a smaller plate can be a handy way to combat the urge to finish everything on our plate, even if we're already full. Of course, if you find that you're hungry too soon after eating a meal, you might need to use a bigger plate. It's just about knowing what you are doing and making changes to suit you.

Once you have identified when, where and what you are eating, you can look at strategies to improve or tweak your diet. I always suggest that clients focus on what to include, rather than what to avoid. Focusing on including means there will be little room for less nutritious foods anyway, and you won't feel deprived. Focusing on which foods to avoid can sometimes backfire. After all, when someone tells you not to jump in that puddle or not to go in that room, what do you automatically want to do?

I remember one lunchtime at Hawthorn I was busy taking players' skinfold measurements, so I asked one of the footballers, Jack Gunston, to bring me lunch from the buffet in the club kitchen. After what seemed like forever, he finally returned. I asked him what had taken him so long and he said, 'You don't know how hard it is to get you lunch. I was under pressure. If I serve you too much, it might give the impression that I think you eat too much. If I don't give you enough, you might think I think you should eat less.' Wow – what a lot of thinking over one plate of food. We should think about what we serve, but try not to overanalyse it to the point that it becomes stressful.

STEP 3. SETTING YOURSELF UP FOR SUCCESS

Healthy eating is not about banning foods; it's about making the healthy choice the easy and desirable one. A fresh, crisp apple is more appealing than a soft, wrinkly one, just as a cut orange is more appealing than a whole one. (Who wants to peel it? It will probably just stay in your lunch box or training bag.) Surrounding yourself with quality, easily prepared, nutritious food choices is an invitation to success.

Try stocking up on:

- » punnets of berries (these might seem expensive, but they don't cost any more than something from the vending machine or coffee shop)
- » fresh nuts (a handful)
- » crackers and tasty cheese
- » trail mix (this can stay in your training bag, as it keeps for weeks).

Choose whatever appeals to you and have it ready to go. All foods are okay sometimes – it's the quantity and frequency that affects your health and performance.

I was recently in the supermarket looking to buy some chocolate when an elderly gentleman stopped and said to me, 'Yes, enjoy some chocolate! Don't listen to what those dietitians say!' I thought he must have been a client of mine having a joke, but I didn't know him. I responded, 'I think it's good to enjoy all foods, even if I am one of those dietitians.' He backpedalled, apologising, and insisted that he wasn't having a go at my profession, he just didn't want to give up certain foods. I reassured him that I don't believe you have to give up any foods to be healthy – just surround yourself with nutritious foods that most of your food intake can come from.

One of my clients found it difficult to break her habit of eating the charity chocolates that sat on her desk at work. Her difficulty was she had limited choice – it was either the chocolate or her piece of fruit, and the chocolate usually won. To turn this around she brought in a variety of fruit, which gave her a choice between her fruits, rather than between her one fruit versus the chocolate. She also focused on how much less sluggish she felt after eating the fruit than the chocolate, and told herself that the chocolates weren't forbidden, and that she could enjoy them occasionally.

An AFL player I worked with was struggling to break the habit of regularly drinking soft drink at home. He found that he would regress whenever visitors came over. To tackle this, he put a sign on his fridge: 'No soft drink in this fridge'. His visitors complained at first, but they soon realised it was important to help him achieve what he wanted, and to support him.

Regular dinners with friends and family can be tricky when you are trying to eat for success. When I first started visiting my Maltese mother-in-law she would serve me a delicious bowl of pasta so large that I would feel like I was going to burst! When others are serving up the meal, guide them on how much you would like. Serve yourself if possible, and don't be scared to leave some on your plate. It's not being rude, it is helping you – you are listening and responding to what your body needs. I learnt to ask for less, as the overeating felt horrible, and I knew I was going to be eating there regularly.

When working with athletes who live away from home during the season and then return home to their families in the off-season, especially at Christmas breaks, I have had to develop strategies for them to politely ask for less food, or ask if they can serve themselves. This can be a particular challenge during celebratory feasts, especially for athletes – people sometimes feel they need to 'feed up' people who are very active. Try and eat until you are comfortable, rather than overeating. It's hard to train when you have overeaten or haven't slept well after eating too much.

GETTING YOUR BALANCE

The amount and type of food we need differs between people, and changes throughout life stages, such as in times of growth (early childhood and teenage years), pregnancy, lactation and older age, as well as varying between active and inactive days and periods of muscle gain or fat loss, illness or injury. The stage you are at will dictate your dietary requirements.

It is possible to get the right balance of macronutrients (the nutrients that provide energy: carbohydrate, fat and protein) within a single meal, but not always. This might balance out over the day, or over a few days. It doesn't have to balance at every meal, nor do you always want it to. Some meals might need to be higher in carbohydrate than others, such as a bowl of pasta before an endurance event or for recovery, and some meals will be higher in protein, such as a steak after a weights session. This will vary according to your individual needs.

The macronutrient balance is often discussed as being around 30 per cent of energy from fat, 20 per cent from protein and 50 per cent from carbohydrate.

In general, for overall health and disease prevention, the recommendation is to cover the dinner plate with around one-quarter each of protein and carbohydrate foods and half a plate of vegetables. For more active people, one-third of each may be more suitable. This visual plate coverage description is much easier and more practical to implement than calculating percentages of energy from each macronutrient.

We know that most Australians don't eat enough vegetables – five or more servings per day is the recommended amount. To improve our dietary balance, we need to include more vegetables. (Many also need to reduce the carbohydrate load, and choose wholegrain varieties.) If we did this it would leave the other half of the plate free to be shared between protein and carbohydrate foods, which would be a good balance for most of us, most of the time. If only it were that simple.

Food rules such as 'no carbohydrates after 5 pm' are an example of trying to reduce carbohydrate intake and control portions and kilojoules, generally in order to achieve weight loss. These kinds of rules focus on what you shouldn't eat, and instil guilt and a feeling of deprivation around food. If pasta is a food you enjoy, are you really never going to eat it after 5 pm again? This is not sustainable for long-term health and food enjoyment, and it's unnecessary. To help achieve balance, think about the other foods you plan to eat throughout the day. Could these have more protein and vegetables, and a little less carbohydrate? With the pasta, would you be happy with a smaller serving size, and a few vegetables on the side instead? Could you include a protein in the pasta sauce, or as dessert afterwards?

To help find your balance, try monitoring yourself and making modifications. Things you can monitor include:

- » how you recover after exercise
- » how you feel during exercise: did you have enough energy, or did you feel sluggish from over- or under-eating? If you felt fast and light, this is an indication that the meal was suited for you.
- » changes in body composition (gain or loss of muscle)
- » health measures – blood sugar (glucose), blood pressure, blood cholesterol levels, hormone levels, bone density, iron

- » frequency of colds and infections (these can be caused by not eating enough, or the timing of food post-exercise)
- » bowel habits (regularity, bloating, microbiome diversity).

Here are a few examples of situations that might be improved or resolved by a change in the macronutrient (carbohydrate, fat and protein) balance:

- » **Muscle mass loss:** Muscle mass can be lost when we are inactive. To help reduce this loss, make sure you are eating enough protein, and spread your protein intake out over the day, rather than having one bulk load in the evening. Breakfast is often a meal that lacks protein. Try adding milk, yoghurt, eggs, legumes or cheese to your breakfast, and maybe have a little less bread or cereal.
- » **Feeling tired when exercising:** Are you consuming enough carbohydrate during the day? Try to include some in each meal, and have some before exercise. Include good-quality wholegrain carbohydrates, such as wholegrain bread, high-fibre breakfast cereal, fruit for snacks, and potatoes, sweet potato or rice with your meal post-exercise, for recovery. Bear in mind that too much carbohydrate, particularly refined varieties, may make you feel lethargic. Experiment a little until you find the right balance for you.
- » **Feeling tired and sluggish after the evening meal:** Increasing the amount of vegetables in your evening meal and reducing the other types of foods might be the key to resolving this. In addition, try eating less overall, so that you are comfortable rather than overfull – you can eat again later if needed. Even when eating healthy foods, it's possible to eat too much. Are you overeating in the evening because you're not eating enough earlier in the day? Are you drinking enough water? Being dehydrated can also make you feel tired.
- » **Blood glucose levels are high mid morning:** For people with diabetes in particular, this could be because your breakfast is packed with carbohydrate and doesn't have enough protein, good fats or fibre in it. Have a piece of wholegrain toast with cheese and tomato instead of wholemeal or white bread with jam. Choose a breakfast cereal with at least 8 grams of dietary fibre per 100 grams, and balance it with some natural yoghurt or milk – the protein in these will slow the rate of

carbohydrate digestion. Eat only until you are comfortable, but not full, and have another snack or meal later if needed. This will help reduce the carbohydrate load you are having at one time.

» **Getting hungry only an hour or so after breakfast:** It might be that you're having a low-fibre carbohydrate for breakfast, which will be digested very quickly, such as white toast and honey or a high-sugar, low-fibre cereal. It might also lack sufficient protein and some healthy fats, both of which will keep you full for longer.

Swap the white toast for a heavy rye or wholegrain bread, or the cereal for some Bircher muesli to increase the fibre. To increase the protein, add a good dollop or two of yoghurt to the cereal, along with a sprinkle of chia seeds and nuts (these contain healthy fats as well), or have a slice of cheese or egg on the toast.

Adding volume and fibre with foods such as mushrooms, tomato, avocado or baked beans will also keep you full for longer. Also consider whether you're eating enough at breakfast – you may need to increase the total amount, particularly if you have completed morning exercise.

TIPS FOR EATING FOR SUCCESS

Whether you're an athlete or not, there are some basic nutritional principles we can all follow to help keep a healthy balance. Here a few general tips:

» Surround yourself with nutritious food choices and have your life influencers (e.g. household members, work colleagues, coaches, training partners) on your side, understanding your needs and willing to support you.

» Include vegetables in meals and snacks – this way there won't be room for many less-nutritious foods. Doing this will also shift your focus to foods to include, rather than those you want to avoid or restrict.

» Look at basic nutrition messages – two fruit, five vegetables, a handful of nuts (~30–50 grams per day) and around three calcium serves (1 serve = 300 milligrams) per day, and consider the importance of quantity and variety of dietary fibre.

» Stop when you're 7/10 full = comfortable.

» Get in tune with your body so you know when you are full, hungry and thirsty. This awareness can guide your serving size at each meal.

» Change the type and amount of food you eat depending on your training needs, rest days, injury, competition days and how you feel. This does not have to be set.

» Choose nutritious foods to satisfy hunger and less nutritious foods in smaller quantities to satisfy desire. For example, when you're starving, don't grab a block of chocolate or you are likely to devour it all. Instead, try a punnet of berries with some yoghurt, or make a sandwich and leave room for a little chocolate to enjoy afterwards. The serving size of chocolate will then be moderate, to please your desire, rather than your hunger, and you will have gained the nutrients you needed as well.

» Cook at home more often. Research shows that people who prepare food at home are more likely to eat smaller portions, take in fewer kilojoules and consume less saturated fat, salt and sugar. This is particularly important when athletes need to 'make weight' and for reducing body fat levels at different times of preparation. The serving size of vegetables at restaurants is usually far too small, unless you are prepared to pay what is often an exorbitant price for a side of greens.

» Make smart food swaps. Focus on wholefoods over packaged and highly processed foods. For example, choose:
  » a tub of natural yoghurt and a bunch of grapes rather than a processed recovery bar
  » a snack pack of sultanas with a stick of cheese in a lunch box instead of chips
  » tuna, a hard-boiled egg or cheese and avocado on wholegrain crackers for an afternoon pre-training snack, instead of sweet biscuits.

Now that we have an idea of what we are doing and what we can do for success, let's get down to the nitty-gritty.

CHAPTER 2
The Carbohydrate Guide

SHOULD I EAT CARBS?

The answer to this question is most definitely yes. This doesn't mean you need to overdo it, of course – balance is still key. Eating a massive bowl of pasta just because you have a match the next day can be excessive. Rather than giving you energy, this is more likely to leave you feeling heavy and bloated and may interrupt your sleep.

WHICH CARBOHYDRATES ARE THE BEST?

There are many different carbohydrate-containing foods. Some are nutrient rich, offering a combination of micronutrients (vitamins and minerals), antioxidants, protein, healthy fats, dietary fibre and/or resistant starch, which is beneficial for gut health (see chapter 9 for more information about this). For example, rice, legumes and pasta contain protein, carbohydrate and an array of micronutrients. Fruit contains carbohydrate, fibre and micronutrients. This range of nutrient-rich carbohydrates is what we should be eating most of for good health.

All plant foods contain varying degrees of carbohydrate: fruits, vegetables, grains and legumes, to a smaller degree seeds and nuts. In the animal world, dairy provides carbohydrate in the form of the sugar lactose.

When it comes to grains, as a general rule, those carbohydrates that are higher in dietary fibre are the ones to choose. We know wholegrains have beneficial effects on health, reducing the risk of chronic diseases such as diabetes, heart disease and some cancers, particularly bowel cancer, which are all major causes of death in Australia. The dietary fibre also helps with good gut health, thus benefiting overall health.

Foods containing high dietary fibre, such as wholemeal pasta, legumes and vegetables, help keep you feeling full for longer. These are particularly useful for those sports with body composition and weight restrictions.

The low-nutrient carbohydrates such as soft drink, sports drinks, lollies, cakes and biscuits should be kept to a minimum, as they offer little nutritional value and can be detrimental to health. These can be beneficial for quick, easily available energy under certain circumstances, such as during endurance events, marathons, long hikes, triathlons and high-intensity exercise lasting longer than 60 minutes.

STRUCTURE OF CARBOHYDRATES AND THE GLYCAEMIC INDEX

Carbohydrates can contain sugars. There are many different types of sugars, including glucose, lactose, galactose, sucrose and starches. Many carbohydrates – often referred to as 'good' or 'complex' carbohydrates – contain starches. Starches are made up of glucose molecules joined together in long chains called polysaccharides. I think of these chains as a string of beads, with each 'bead' being a glucose molecule. These molecules are digested, ready to be absorbed into the bloodstream.

These polysaccharide chains can be made up of either amylose or amylopectin starches. An amylose chain is one straight chain, while an amylopectin chain has numerous branches. Foods with a greater proportion of amylopectin starch are digested more quickly, because those branches are easily accessible to the digestive enzymes that break down the polysaccharide chains.

We can measure how rapidly a carbohydrate-containing food is digested and how much glucose is released into the bloodstream. This measurement is known as the glycaemic index (GI) rating for that food. Carbohydrates that are high in amylopectin are generally higher in GI, for example, white bread, short-grain rice, sushi rice and many low-fibre breakfast cereals.

The release of glucose into the bloodstream triggers your pancreas to release the hormone insulin. The insulin picks up the glucose from the bloodstream and takes it into muscle, liver and fat cells to use later. Too much insulin can promote fat storage.

The lower the GI, the more gradual the release of carbohydrate, and therefore the release of energy. Lower-GI foods may also keep you full for longer. This is why they are often considered to be more desirable, particularly for those aiming for weight reduction. However, a low GI rating is not a guarantee that a food is necessarily nutritious. For example, highly processed, low-nutrient-containing foods such as doughnuts and potato crisps are high in carbohydrate and have a relatively low GI. The high fat content slows the rate of digestion, and this is what lowers the GI. Nutrient-rich foods such as pineapple, grapes and mashed potatoes have a higher GI rating but offer an array of valuable nutrients, so would be more nutritious choices.

Sometimes people tell me they have stopped eating potatoes and swapped them for sweet potato, because sweet potato has a lower GI. The poor humble spud! There is no need to avoid potato. Foods are usually eaten as a meal, and the GI becomes a combination of all the foods in the meal, along with the amount of the food eaten. Protein and fat will help lower the overall GI, so, for example, if you are eating your potatoes with meat, the GI will be lowered. It also depends on how the food has been cooked. A roasted or mashed sweet potato will have a higher GI than a boiled one.

Knowing the glycaemic index of foods can be useful when choosing what to eat during and immediately after exercise. Higher GI foods can be preferable in the following situations:

- » During exercise, higher GI foods are best if fuel is needed quickly during the event.
- » Post-exercise, higher GI foods will start replenishing carbohydrate stores more quickly.
- » In between sessions, especially if another session is not far away, eat higher GI foods to replenish carbohydrate stores. This means the food will be digested more quickly, and won't be sitting in your stomach during the next session. The food will also give you energy for the session.

There are many different scenarios in which a high or low GI food, or a combination of both, might be useful. Remember, the GI of a carbohydrate food is affected by the foods eaten with it. The most important thing to consider is the overall nutritional content of the food.

HOW MUCH CARBOHYDRATE DO I NEED?

It can be easy to overindulge on many carbohydrate foods. Whole grains, rather than processed grains, have the dietary fibre to fill you up more. They also take longer to eat, as you need to chew them more, which slows you down a little.

Determining your carbohydrate needs can be tricky, as requirements vary for each individual, and can also vary from day to day. I have included a guide below, but bear in mind that most of us do not need to start counting – there are other strategies we can use to estimate our carbohydrate intake.

A GUIDE TO YOUR CARBOHYDRATE NEEDS

- Sedentary–low-intensity exercise: 3–5 grams of carbohydrate per kilogram of body weight
- Moderate-intensity exercise, daily for 1 hour: 5–7 grams of carbohydrate per kilogram of body weight
- Moderate–high-intensity exercise for 1–3 hours per day: 6–10 grams of carbohydrate per kilogram of body weight
- High intensity–ironman/ultra-endurance athletes, 15+ hours training per week: 10–12 grams of carbohydrate per kilogram of body weight

Personally, I don't enjoy counting any aspect of my food. I am moderately active, so I don't need to count grams of carbohydrate per day. Around a quarter of the volume of my food needs to come from carbohydrate – up to a third on more active days. I look at the proportions I am serving. I cover around half of the plate or bowl with non-starchy vegetables, and a quarter each with protein and carbohydrate foods. If I am eating a bowl of pasta or risotto my high-carbohydrate food is half or more for that meal, but things balance out over time – the next night I may eat a steak and salad, and no or only a small serve of potato. The protein and vegetables are greater in that meal, and the carbohydrate less. Listening to my body, paying attention to how I feel and my energy levels, and adjusting my carbohydrate intake accordingly works for me.

If your training is more demanding, and you are completing heavy training sessions on some days, plan to have your higher-carbohydrate meals before and after these sessions, and the lower-carbohydrate meals on your rest days. Listen to what your body wants. If you are extra hungry and feel like you need more energy, serve yourself an extra scoop or two of mashed potato or rice. If you feel like a bowl of pasta, go for it. Just eat until you're comfortable, not until you need to be rolled away from the table.

Spreading your carbohydrate intake out over the day is generally better than having one large serving, particularly if you are wanting to gain muscle mass and body weight. Eating enough total kilojoules is very important for this. The carbohydrate kilojoules replenish muscle glycogen and energy, leaving the protein for building muscle.

For endurance events, carbohydrate intake may need to be increased days before an event. It can be a mistake to overeat carbohydrates the night before intense exercise such as a football, rugby, soccer or netball game, thinking you need to carbohydrate load extensively. Eating too much carbohydrate can make you feel sluggish and can affect your sleep. As carbohydrate stores water with it, too much can make you feel heavy and slow.

CARBOHYDRATE CONTENT OF SOME NUTRITIOUS FOOD CHOICES	
FOOD	CARBOHYDRATE CONTENT (GRAMS)
1 slice bread (30 g – weights vary greatly)	15
Wholemeal pasta (100 g dry)	66
1 corn cob (100 g)	16
Brown rice (100 g cooked)	23
White potato (100 g boiled)	20
Sweet potato (100 g boiled)	20
Pumpkin (100 g boiled)	7
Wheat biscuits breakfast cereal (2 biscuits)	22
Rolled oats (½ cup raw)	25
Banana (1 medium)	20
Strawberries (½ cup)	6
Grapes (½ cup)	12
Milk 2% fat (1 cup, 250 ml)	12.5
Kidney beans (100 g cooked)	9
Baked beans, canned, flavoured (140 g)	19

HAVE YOU TRIED ANCIENT GRAINS?

In Western society we are just discovering numerous grains that many other societies have been cooking as staples for years. These 'ancient grains' are becoming popular due to their high nutritional value.

Ancient grains tend to be less processed (the husk is left on), which is nutritionally better for us. The husk increases the fibre content, protein level and some vitamins and minerals, such as manganese, selenium and magnesium. This wholegrain nature also means the grains require more chewing, which helps us slow down our eating and stop before we are too full.

Including ancient grains in your diet increases the range of nutritious carbohydrate sources you have to choose from, which is particularly great for very active people who need lots of carbohydrates. Including a variety of plant forms in your diet is the key to getting a great range of nutrients.

EXAMPLES OF ANCIENT GRAINS

- » **Freekeh:** wheat that is harvested when young and green, then toasted and cracked. Being young, freekeh has a higher nutrient content than mature wheat. It is also high in fibre, containing four times more fibre than brown rice. Some of this fibre is resistant starch, meaning it can't be digested in the small intestine, so it passes to your large intestine, where it becomes food for good gut bacteria.

  Freekeh also contains minerals such as magnesium, selenium, iron, zinc, copper and potassium. It has a low GI, so will only gradually raise your blood glucose levels. This makes it great for people who have diabetes, and perfect for providing sustaining energy throughout the day. Try it in a salad for lunch, or in a stir-fry instead of white rice if you'll be training later in the day.

» **Quinoa:** the best-known of these ancient grains, although it is not actually a grain itself. Quinoa is related to the beet and spinach family. It's the seed of the quinoa plant that we eat.

Quinoa is interesting because it has a higher protein content than rice or pasta. It has twice the protein of rice, and also contains all nine essential amino acids, making it a complete protein, unlike other plant grains. That is particularly good news for people following vegetarian and vegan diets. It also has a great range of B-group vitamins.

Quinoa is high in soluble fibre, which is great for lowering cholesterol and keeping the bowels regular. It is also gluten free. It comes in white, red and black varieties. Although it can be expensive compared to other alternatives, eating quinoa is a great way to add variety to your diet. It works well in salads, and in hot dishes.

» **Amaranth:** tiny seeds that are used like a grain, but are not actually classified as a grain. Amaranth is higher in protein, iron and calcium than wheat, and can be boiled or made into a flour. It is gluten free and high in dietary fibre. It contains around 6 per cent fat, and these are mostly unsaturated fats. Most amaranth available in Australia is imported.

» **Barley:** a cereal grain that is usually processed to make pearl barley, which is produced by removing the two outer layers. Barley is not gluten free, but it is lower in gluten than wheat. That's why barley isn't often used in bread making, or only in small amounts – the gluten is what gives the dough elasticity.

Barley contains a compound called beta-glucan (also found in oats), which benefits cholesterol and heart health. Barley, because the husk has been left on, is also high in dietary fibre and contains a range of vitamins, minerals and antioxidants. The CSIRO has developed a barley strain called BARLEYmax (GM free) that is particularly high in dietary fibre, including resistant starch, which is important for bowel health, and beta-glucan, which helps reduce cholesterol levels. BARLEYmax can be found in a range of foods.

» **Teff:** seeds that are around the size of a poppy seed. Because teff is so small, it is eaten whole and unprocessed. It is boiled like you would rice, but takes less time to cook. It can be ground into flour to make sourdough breads such as injera, which is traditional to Ethiopia. Teff is used in numerous gluten-free products. It contains more calcium than other grains – around 123 milligrams to 1 cup cooked.

» **Spelt:** a subspecies of wheat. Spelt has had a recent resurgence in popularity, as it is lower in fructan (a fermentable carbohydrate) than standard wheat. This provides some relief to people who are wheat intolerant or wheat sensitive. However, it is not suitable for those with coeliac disease, as it still contains gluten. We will talk more about these fermentable carbohydrates in the chapter on gut health (see page 93).

Cooking with spelt means you can still enjoy the taste, texture and health benefits of a wholegrain wheat bread or pasta.

WHAT ABOUT SUGAR?

Sugar is a carbohydrate, and too much sugar isn't ideal. However, it should not be totally demonised:

- » Our brains run on the simplest form of sugar: glucose.
- » Our muscles store glucose as glycogen and then use it to produce ATP (adenosine triphosphate) for muscle contraction.
- » Glucose can provide immediate energy for those times when you need to accelerate, such as when you need to sprint at the end of a race. Carbohydrate is what provides the immediate energy required.
- » Sugar does make many foods taste better, and it is okay to eat food because it tastes good. It's the quantity and frequency of this that will affect your health.

Sugars are a class of carbohydrates that contain oxygen hydrogen groups (OH), found in animals and plants, and that have a sweet taste. Common sugars are glucose, sucrose, fructose and lactose. Sucrose is the most common form of sugar. Sucrose is commonly used to sweeten tea and coffee, and in baking. This is the sugar you buy by the kilogram (white, brown or raw). Sucrose's molecular structure is one fructose and one glucose molecule joined together.

Sucrose is commonly found in highly processed foods with added sugar and minimal nutrients, often called 'empty' calorie foods. These include soft drink, cordial, energy drinks, sports drinks, lollies, some bars, biscuits, and low-fibre, high-sugar breakfast cereals. These foods give us energy (calories or kilojoules) from carbohydrate without providing any other nutrients. These should be limited in a daily diet.

When training for more than 90 minutes and during competitions, the high-sugar, lower-fibre foods may be appropriate, because the body wants carbohydrate quickly. These foods are easy to eat, and rapidly release the carbohydrate into the bloodstream. However, these foods should be consumed minimally, as excess sugar is not beneficial to our health.

If participating in an endurance event such as an iron man competition or a marathon, increasing your carbohydrate intake a few days prior to competing helps increase your body's glycogen stores. Foods containing added sugar can be helpful to meet the carbohydrate requirements of endurance athletes, which may be up to 10 grams of carbohydrate per kilogram of body weight when carbohydrate loading.

Great, easy-to-eat options to top up energy stores or refuel pre- or post-exercise include adding honey to cereal (note: honey is high in fructose, which can cause gastric upsets to those who are fructose intolerant), drinking a sports drink (note that there is no nutritional value in this choice apart from water and sugar) or flavoured milk (the milk is a healthy choice, the flavouring is the low-nutrient sugar part), and eating yoghurt and custard that contains added sugar, a muesli bar or a lower-fibre breakfast cereal with added sugar.

When the activity is high intensity and greater than 90–120 minutes, it can be beneficial to top up carbohydrate stores with a combination of sugar types. Consuming glucose and fructose together results in more rapid emptying of carbohydrate from the intestine, as each type uses a different transporter. Maximising carbohydrate uptake in this way is referred to as having multiple transportable carbohydrates. Including both sugar types therefore helps delay the onset of fatigue.

If your muscles run out of stored glycogen and there is no carbohydrate intake from food or fluid to provide more, muscles will take glucose from the blood, resulting in a reduction in blood glucose levels. To continue, your exercise intensity will be forced to drop – this is known as 'hitting the wall'. Hence, carbohydrate is very important to being able to sustain the high intensity.

Playing sport or exercising for an hour or so is not a reason to eat a pile of lollies. There are much better choices of carbohydrate-containing foods that also contain other valuable nutrients – for example, fruit. With all the sports teams I have worked with, I've stopped lollies being handed out post-game. During the game a few lollies can provide easily digested carbohydrate. But post-game, it's important to consume carbohydrate food sources that will also replace some protein, vitamins, minerals and antioxidants for overall repair. Foods such as rice pudding, chicken wraps, risotto, lean meat burgers, fruit and milk are all popular choices. At this point players may also drink some sports drink to aid with replacing carbohydrates, electrolytes and water. The players are physically exhausted at this time, so liquid replacement of nutrients is appealing.

FRUCTOSE

Fructose is a sugar (carbohydrate) naturally found in fruit, fruit juice, some vegetables, syrups (such as maple syrup) and honey. It has had some bad publicity, with critics linking dietary fructose with obesity, high triglyceride (blood fat) levels and insulin resistance. The body processes fructose differently to other sugars, which is why there seems to be a concern.

Fructose, like glucose, is digested and transported to the liver. The difference is that glucose relies on the hormone insulin to release it for use by cells, whereas fructose does not require insulin. This means there are two possible ways of sugar absorption. Some sports gels and drinks will contain both glucose and fructose for this reason.

We don't really know whether fructose acts differently when found naturally in a food, like fruit, compared to when it has been refined into a syrup and added to a processed food such as a biscuit or a drink. What we do know is that most Australians are eating and drinking too much total sugar, and we need to reduce that amount. Reducing our intake of foods containing fructose syrups, which are often low-nutrient-containing foods, will reduce our total sugar intake.

We know that the fructose found naturally in our fruit and vegetables is not in a concentrated form, and provides overall nutritional benefits. These foods should be thoroughly enjoyed, and only limited if gut issues (such as fructose malabsorption – see page 109) occur.

HOW MUCH SUGAR IS TOO MUCH?

There is a lot of talk about sugar being the root of the growing prevalence of obesity. Sugar may be a contributing factor, but we can't blame one nutrient alone. We need to look at our whole diet, and our lifestyles, too.

The 2011–12 Australian Health Survey showed that Australians were eating, on average, 60 grams – about 14 teaspoons, or 10.95 per cent of total energy intake – of free sugars a day. A free sugar is one that is added to foods in processing, also found in honey, syrups and the natural or added sugars in fruit juice. This figure is an average, which means that many people are eating larger amounts. As a population, we need to look at cutting down on our added sugar intake.

The World Health Organization (WHO) recommends cutting free sugars to less than 10 per cent of total energy (or kilojoule) intake – preferably to 5 per cent for additional health benefits. For an adult eating the average of 8700 kilojoules a day (this is the average used by the Australian Dietary Guidelines when making dietary recommendations), this means no more than 51 grams, which is about 13 teaspoons a day, and ideally 25 grams or 6–7 teaspoons. This recommendation is referring to the added sugars in foods and drinks, not the sugar found naturally in your fruit, vegetables and milk.

The Australian Dietary Guidelines specifically recommend limiting intake of foods containing added sugars, such as confectionery, soft drink, fruit drinks, cordial, vitamin waters, energy drinks, sports drinks, biscuits and cakes.

Reading food labels can help you to identify where you are consuming sugar in your diet. Ingredients that end in 'ose' are usually a type of sugar, such as glucose, fructose, dextrose, glucose syrups and maltose. Ingredients such as rice syrups, concentrated fruit juice, honey, sugar (this is 50:50 glucose and fructose), and palm sugar are also sugars. A total avoidance of sugar is unnecessary, but many of us should cut down, even if we are active.

The confusion many have with sugar and sugar content was clearly illustrated when I met a keen cyclist at a flavoured milk launch. I was there to discuss the nutritional benefits of milk, particularly in sports nutrition. The cyclist told me he adds 30 grams of glucose to his protein powder and water mix post-workouts. However, he said he would never drink flavoured milk for his recovery because of the sugar content. What he, along with many people, didn't know is that glucose is pure sugar. Sugar comes in lots of different forms, and he was consuming it in its simplest form: glucose.

Glucose is absorbed by the body more quickly than any other sugar, as it is in a form ready to be absorbed. This is useful if blood glucose levels have dropped dangerously low, or when a person needs to replenish glycogen stores as quickly as possible, but this man was going to sit at his desk for the rest of the day, and had 24 hours to replenish before his next session. He told me the people he trained with had recommended this. It amazes me that people eat and drink foods, and sometimes even take supplements, without questioning what they are putting into their bodies. This cyclist, who wanted to avoid sugar, was giving himself a large dose after every workout – and spending dollars doing it.

WHAT ABOUT FRUIT?

Australians are not eating enough fruit. The most recent Australian Health Survey in 2011–12 found that just 52 per cent of Australians meet the recommendation of two servings of fruit per day for adults.

Fruit contains a mix of glucose and fructose (the proportions vary). Some people get concerned about this sugar, but they shouldn't. Two servings of fruit is a good guide for nutritional benefits, and can be increased for those with greater energy needs. It wouldn't be unusual for the footballers I work with to eat four pieces of fruit per day – one at breakfast on their cereal, one with lunch, one as part of an afternoon snack and one with yoghurt for dessert.

Fruit is an economical, accessible, sweet snack, and most of us like some sweetness. I have plenty of clients who are concerned about the number of fruit servings they should have in a day due to the sugar content. But if you are hungry I wouldn't want you to say, 'I've already had my two serves of fruit today so I'll have some potato chips now' – that would be ridiculous! Listen to your body and enjoy these nutritious foods. If your energy needs are greater, eat more fruit every day. You might eat three serves one day, and one the next.

The Australian Dietary Guidelines are based on an average person with a requirement of 8700 kilojoules per day, but if you are exercising most days at a moderate to intense rate, your energy requirements will probably be greater. Eating fruit would be a great way to get some of those extra kilojoules. I could eat loads of my father-in-law's homegrown peaches. If he let me, I would park myself under the tree and eat them all day long.

When eating dried fruit, just remember that, for example, one dried apricot is equivalent in sugar to a whole apricot – only the water has been removed. Dried fruits are concentrated sources of sugars, and it's easy to go overboard with them. However, snacking on dried fruit is a great way to top up carbohydrate stores when you are travelling. The little boxes of sultanas you can buy are a handy nutritious sweet food to have in your lunchbox or on your desk, and a perfect top-up pre-, during or post-training. My daughter loves dried mango. Given her sweet tooth, I'd prefer she have a piece of dried mango rather than biscuits or lollies, which I know she would be eating otherwise. Dried fruit has the added bonus of providing vitamins, minerals, antioxidants and dietary fibre, and it tastes good. Just bear in mind that the dietary fibre content of dried fruit means it can have a laxative effect, and it is a concentrated form of fructose that can cause gastrointestinal bloating for some people. Find your tolerance limits.

WHAT ABOUT FRUIT JUICE?

Fruit juice contains around the same amount of sugar as soft drink – 10 per cent – so a 250 millilitre glass contains around 25 grams of sugar. When fruit juices are made, the flesh and skin of the fruit is generally taken out, meaning the dietary fibre has been removed. This is the part that's great for our bowels and helps fill us up with minimal kilojoules/calories. Once we pulp fruit into juice we're left with a concentrated form of kilojoules and sugar. If you want to drink juice, the Australian Dietary Guidelines recommend limiting it to 125 millilitres per day, or half a cup.

It can be lovely to have a cold glass of juice. Just drink it slowly, and savour the taste. If you need a carbohydrate boost before or after training, or you need extra kilojoules to help you gain weight, a glass of juice might be a perfect inclusion in your daily dietary intake. A glass of juice with breakfast can be an easy way for young growing athletes to increase kilojoule intake (energy), and on the flip side, reducing juice is an easy way to reduce kilojoule and sugar (energy) intake.

Vegetable-based juices contain less sugar and plenty of nutrients. I recommend a maximum of one serving of fruit to sweeten the drink – the rest should be vegetables, preferably including the pulp. My tip is to lay out the ingredients on a plate before you make your juice. If it is more than you would eat in one sitting, then it is more than you need in one drink – unless you need extra kilojoules, carbohydrates, or a vitamin and mineral boost because you don't eat your veggies.

My daughter often worries that I might pull someone out of the queue at a juice bar and ask if they know what they're about to drink. Do they realise that a 600 millilitre fruit juice will contain around 10–12 per cent sugar? That's 60 grams of sugar in one drink. Adding vegetables will reduce the sugar content, but often there are two or three servings of fruit along with the vegetables. It's easy to 'drink kilojoules' and fall into the trap of replacing more energy than you use during exercise.

TIPS FOR CUTTING BACK ON SUGAR

- Steer clear of soft drink, energy drinks and cordial (they don't offer any nutritional benefit apart from water and sugar). They contain around 10 per cent sugar, and are usually drunk in addition to food. A few exceptions where a high-sugar drink is useful is when fuel reserves need topping up during periods of intense physical activity (more than 60 minutes' duration) or for recovery, when sick and eating minimally, or to counteract low blood sugar levels in people with diabetes.
- Swap lollies and biscuits for a square or two of dark chocolate, fruit (e.g. a punnet of berries) or savoury foods like nuts, wholegrain crackers with cheese, or antipasto (e.g. olives, sundried tomatoes, pickled onions). Don't kid yourself that you need a continual supply of lollies between events – go back to the traditional half-time oranges or a banana. They are perfect. A sandwich cut into quarters and spread out through the day will also do just fine.
- Cut smaller pieces of cake with minimal icing.
- If you drink fruit juice, choose a variety that's 100 per cent fruit juice. Just half a glass (125 millilitres) might be enough.
- Cut down on the amount of sugar you add to tea and coffee.
- Read food labels and look out for words like glucose, glucose syrup, fructose syrup, concentrated fruit juice, honey, rice syrup, and most words that end in 'ose', as these are all types of sugar.

> » Swap ice cream and icy poles for frozen bananas with the tip dipped in dark chocolate. Frozen whole fruit (frozen grapes taste like sherbet bombs) and orange segments are also refreshing.
> » Have a scoop of ice cream in a bowl, rather than numerous spoonfuls eaten straight from the container. Grate on some chocolate instead of having a thickly coated chocolate ice cream on a stick.
> » Make it easy on yourself and buy fewer high-sugar, low-nutrient foods. If they're not in the cupboard or fridge, they're easier to avoid. Stock up on nutrient-rich foods and have them ready to go.

I first started working with the Western Bulldogs in 1994. Back then it was more common to drink sports drinks and eat lollies for quick energy after a game than in recent years. These days, people are more aware of being able to get the carbohydrates they need for recovery and energy from wholefoods, which also provide other nutrients for optimal health and recovery. When I got rid of the lollies near the change rooms, the Hawthorn players weren't pleased. I explained that just a few more steps got them to the kitchen, where they could choose foods that would replace carbohydrates as well as providing other nutrients, such as fruit, a glass of milk or a sandwich. After all, we are looking at maximising performance. The same principle applies for those who are not competing at an elite level. We still want the food we eat to maximise our performance and health.

THE 3 PM ENERGY SLUMP

Do you often find yourself searching for sugar around 3 pm? Our body tends to want to snooze in the afternoon (look at countries that have siestas), so around this time we often want a sugar fix for a quick pick-me-up. The urge will pass, but it helps to be prepared, so try and fuel yourself with nutritious choices instead. Have a container of food ready to grab, such as:

- frozen fruit like berries, mango or pineapple are all great for summer – keep a pack at work in the freezer
- fresh punnets of berries, cherry tomatoes, slices of any kind of melon
- nuts
- hummus or tzatziki dip with cut-up capsicum or carrot and wholegrain crackers
- plain popcorn
- small homemade muffins (add seeds, nuts, yoghurt, oats, fruit, or have savoury muffins with grated vegetables and cheese)
- fruit loaf – sourdough or wholegrain varieties are best
- cheese and biscuits
- wholegrain crackers with peanut butter and sultanas or sliced apple
- milk smoothie.

Having a snack on hand also reduces the chances of:

- raiding the fridge before dinner is cooked
- overeating at dinner because you are so hungry
- grabbing takeaway because you are too hungry to wait and make dinner
- feeling lethargic during an afternoon or early evening exercise session due to lack of fuel.

WHAT FUEL DO I NEED FOR AN AFTERNOON TRAINING SESSION?

Commencing exercise after work, around 5 pm, when you haven't eaten since lunchtime, means you are likely to feel fatigued. To get the best out of your session, you need to go into it feeling like you have prepared and your body has the energy it needs to perform. An hour or two before the session, top up with some protein, carbohydrate and of course fluid. A tub of yoghurt or a handful of nuts and a piece of fresh fruit, a bowl of minestrone soup or some cut-up vegetables, a couple of crackers and a slice of cheese are all great options. The amount of carbohydrate needed will depend on your goals and the duration of your session. A brisk 45-minute walk doesn't require carbohydrate prior – a small snack to curb the hunger is probably all that is needed.

If the session is going to be an intense 60 minutes or more and you want to gain muscle mass, then a smoothie with milk, a piece of fruit, a few tablespoons of yoghurt and a sprinkle of pepitas or other seeds might be needed. Or you might have a second lunch around 3 pm with a toasted tuna or cheese, tomato, avocado and spinach sandwich or two. Note that each of these suggestions includes some carbohydrate, protein and plant foods. Each individual will require different amounts.

CAN I EAT CARBOHYDRATES IN THE EVENING?

Some people think they should avoid carbohydrates altogether in their evening meal, particularly if they want to reduce their body weight or body fat levels. However, this is not necessary. It is about matching carbohydrate intake to your individual needs. If you train in the afternoon or early evening, it is important to include carbohydrate foods in the evening meal in order to replace energy, particularly if you are backing it up with another session first thing in the morning.

Avoid being starving at dinnertime. It can be easy to arrive home hungry and throw together a bowl of pasta or rice, eat it in a rush, hardly chewing, then lay back and realise you're uncomfortably full. Any reduction in body weight from not eating carbohydrate in the evening is mostly due to the overall reduction in kilojoules being eaten, rather than the timing. Reducing carbohydrate intake at any meal may have positive effects on hormones such as insulin and on reducing blood glucose levels that may be high – this is not just related to eating carbohydrates in the evening. Weight loss is likely to occur rapidly due to a reduction in carbohydrate intake, but it is important to consider whether this is sustainable and appropriate for your training needs. Some of this weight loss is also due to fluid loss, as carbohydrate stores water with it in our cells. You could achieve similar weight loss results if you had a meal that included a smaller serving of carbohydrate, more vegetables, some healthy fats and protein. The weight reduction might take slightly longer, but is likely to be more sustainable and enjoyable, and the food will fuel you for exercise more effectively. It can be advantageous to reduce the serving size of carbohydrate-containing foods, but it is not necessary to remove them altogether.

Balance is the key – you don't need strict rules, and you don't need to cut out food groups altogether. The amount of carbohydrate needed on different days and at different meals will vary.

LOW-CARBOHYDRATE, HIGH-FAT DIETS

Some people follow a low-carbohydrate, high-fat diet in order to achieve weight loss, athletic performance benefits or to treat medical conditions, but is this way of eating really beneficial? A low-carbohydrate, high-fat diet (LCHF) is one in which more than 60 per cent of daily energy intake comes from fat and less than 20 per cent comes from carbohydrate. The Australian Dietary Guidelines recommend that around 30 per cent of total energy should come from fat and 50 per cent from carbohydrate. Protein intake provides around 20 per cent of energy intake, both in the LCHF diet and according to the Australian Dietary Guidelines. An extremely low-carbohydrate diet, known as the ketogenic diet, requires an intake of 50 grams or less of carbohydrate per day. This should only be done under medical supervision.

Our body fat stores provide the body with a potentially unlimited reserve of fuel. Having a low-carbohydrate, high-fat diet aims to use some of this fuel reserve and increase the muscles' ability to metabolise fat for energy. The muscles, however, are limited in how much fat they can burn, particularly during high-intensity training. During low-energy-intensity activity, such as walking, most of the energy provided by the body is through fat oxidation. As intensity increases, energy is provided by both fat and carbohydrate. The proportion of energy coming from carbohydrate increases as intensity increases.

Some studies have shown that following a LCHF diet may result in an adaptation in the muscle that enables it to burn more fat. This can be potentially beneficial for an endurance event. However, there is insufficient evidence to suggest that this leads to an improvement in performance. This could be because the higher fat intake may cause an increase in oxygen demand during exercise – oxidising fat for energy uses more oxygen – negatively affecting power output.

We need stored carbohydrate for quick energy release in the muscles. Carbohydrate is the body's preferred energy source for moderate and high-intensity activity. When following a low-carbohydrate diet, your muscle and liver glycogen stores will be lower. These stores are needed to give immediate energy. Imagine you ride 100 kilometres or more and need to sprint to the finish. Your body needs carbohydrate in the muscle to give it a boost, but it isn't there. Would eating some carbohydrate have got you across the line? There are many different thoughts on this approach, and more research needs to be done.

I have often found that people think they are following a LCHF diet, but when we look closely at what they are eating, it turns out they're not. They are unaware that dairy foods, vegetables, legumes and quinoa, for example, all contain varying degrees of carbohydrate, which may be sufficient to top up their carbohydrate stores, maintaining performance.

When people make positive dietary changes, they see improvements in health and performance. Changes such as cutting out less-nutritious carbohydrate foods, soft drink, confectionery and white bread, reducing serving sizes of pasta and white rice, and increasing lower-carbohydrate vegetables that are high in nutrients and antioxidants make a positive difference. These changes can be made while following a LCHF diet, but they can also occur when including some wholegrain carbohydrates and more moderate amounts of healthy fats in the diet.

Studies have shown that people with impaired blood glucose levels benefit from a reduction in carbohydrate intake and an increase in healthy fats. However, it is not necessary to have the fat intake at 60 per cent of energy or the carbohydrate less than 20 per cent to see positive changes. Working with an accredited practising dietitian can assist you in finding what works for you.

CARBOHYDRATE PERIODISATION

Carbohydrate needs will vary, both between individuals and from day to day. Changing your carbohydrate intake around to meet your needs is referred to as periodising your carbohydrate intake – having a higher carbohydrate intake before certain training sessions, and a lower intake before others.

By training with low carbohydrate stores ('training low') for a few sessions a week, it is thought that you may be able to teach your body to burn more fat and spare muscle glycogen (carbohydrate reserves). The idea is that when you then compete, you make sure you have fully stocked carbohydrate stores, and it is suggested you will burn both fat and carbohydrate efficiently. Further research is being conducted in this area to see whether periodisation results in performance improvement.

Sometimes reducing your carbohydrate intake on days when you are less active or before lighter training sessions, when a high carbohydrate intake is not required, can assist with managing body composition.

If a sport has a weight category or there is a requirement to be very lean, then total energy intake sometimes needs to be reduced. It is then important to select which training sessions you will need more carbohydrate for (harder training sessions) and which you can have less for (lighter sessions). Experiment and see what suits you. An accredited sports dietitian can help you work this out.

CHAPTER 3
Protein

Protein is made up of long chains of amino acids. The body digests these chains into individual amino acids, which are absorbed via the digestive tract. They are then joined back together to build proteins as the body needs them.

Our body uses twenty different amino acids, nine of which are essential (histidine, isoleucine, leucine, lysine, methionine, phenylalanine, threonine, tryptophan and valine). These essential amino acids must come from the protein in our diet, as our body cannot make them. We can, however, produce the remaining eleven amino acids – it's a bit like building with Lego blocks, but using hydrogen, carbon and nitrogen atoms instead. The body is continually breaking down and rebuilding proteins – this is called protein turnover. To build more muscle, we need our body to do more making than breaking.

HOW MUCH PROTEIN DO I NEED?

The Australian Recommended Daily Intake (RDI) for protein is:

- » 0.75–1 gram per kilogram of body weight for the average adult
- » 1–1.2 grams per kilogram of body weight during pregnancy and lactation
- » 1.5–1.8 grams per kilogram of body weight for adults with extra requirements, such as heavy training loads, wanting to increase muscle mass, illnesses, wound repair, or people aged 70+ years.

There's some discussion and research suggesting that these recommendations may be too low, as they are set at the minimum intake of protein needed to offset deficiency. An athlete who is looking to maximise performance will have greater protein needs. That said, many of us eat more than the RDI each day.

Research by Professor Stuart Phillips indicates that active people over the age of 40 years need 1.6–2 grams of protein per kilogram of body weight. Dr Phillips suggests spreading the intake of protein out over four or five eating occasions per day, at a rate of 0.3–0.4 grams of protein per kilogram of body weight. For those aged 80+ years, a minimum of 2 grams of protein per kilogram of body weight is recommended. There is good research indicating that 20–30 grams per meal is a good amount of protein, and an easier measure to use than calculating per kilogram of body weight.

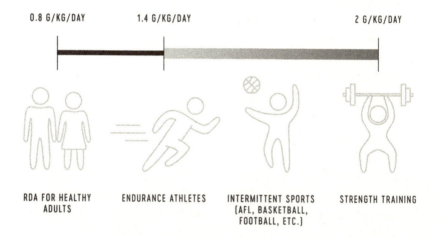

According to the RDI, a person weighing 70 kilograms needs 52.5–70 grams of protein per day. A more active person would need 105–126 grams of protein per day.

We all need to maintain our muscle mass – not just athletes. That is why being active, combined with eating a good diet, can be so powerful. We should aim for an optimal protein intake, rather than just consuming enough to offset deficiency. It is important to look at how you spread your protein intake out over the day. Aim to include 20–25 grams of protein at each meal or snack for muscle repair and growth. Some individuals, particularly heavier people and those undertaking strength training, might need to increase this to 30 grams of protein in order to reach their daily total. Some meals will contain more protein than this, and that's fine, as long as the minimum has been reached and the daily target is met and the protein is not in excessive amounts.

WHEN SHOULD I EAT MY PROTEIN?

Protein is just one part of your diet, and the balance of your overall diet is important. Try to mostly eat meals or snacks that contain protein as well as carbohydrate, vegetables and healthy fats. Spreading protein out over the day is recommended for a few reasons:

1. The body can only use a certain amount of protein at one time for muscle protein synthesis. The rest is broken down to glucose and either used for energy or stored. The nitrogen part of the protein structure is removed, and excreted as urea in urine. Some excess protein may move into the large intestine where bacteria ferment it. Research is investigating whether too much protein in the large intestine may cause gut lining damage.

2. When it comes to muscle mass maintenance and growth, we want our body to be in an anabolic (building) state rather than a catabolic (breaking down) state. Supplying protein regularly (around four or five times in a day) can help stimulate this.

3. Protein helps with satiety (keeping you full for longer), which is helpful for weight management. This can be important in many sports, such as weight category sports, long-distance running and even AFL, where players need to keep lean and strong, and not too bulky.

4. Protein also lowers the glycaemic index of a meal (if carbohydrates are eaten with it), resulting in a more gradual release of the carbohydrate. Having a balance of protein and carbohydrate, rather than a large carbohydrate meal, helps with blood sugar control, as the carbohydrate load is reduced. This also reduces the amount of insulin that is released. You may have heard about insulin resistance, which is related to some health issues such as diabetes, and makes weight reduction difficult. A balance between carbohydrate and protein assists with this.

It can be tricky to have 20–25 grams of protein at breakfast, especially if your breakfast is just a cup of tea and a slice of toast. A 250 millilitre glass of milk gives around 10 grams of protein, and a bowl of cereal provides around 3 grams. After the overnight fast, it is important to eat some protein with breakfast to help maintain muscle mass.

WAYS TO BOOST YOUR PROTEIN AT BREAKFAST

- milk on cereal (read the label for protein content), as well as yoghurt
- rice pudding with added nuts and seeds and quark yoghurt
- Bircher muesli
- chia pudding (with cow's milk or soy for sufficient protein)
- smoothie made with milk and yoghurt (look for higher protein choices)
- breakfast burrito with beans, cheese and vegetables
- eggs, either poached, scrambled, boiled or as an omelette
- frittata, quiche
- beans – kidney, canned baked beans, hummus
- tuna, salmon, smoked salmon, sardines or herrings on toast or with eggs and vegetables
- spreads and additions of sides such as nut spread, cheese, cottage, quark, ricotta or feta cheese
- higher-protein breads, which contain lentils and legumes

THE POWER OF PROTEIN: MUSCLE GROWTH

Eating more protein does not automatically result in greater muscle growth. Physical activity, plus the right nutrition, equals muscle repair, maintenance and growth.

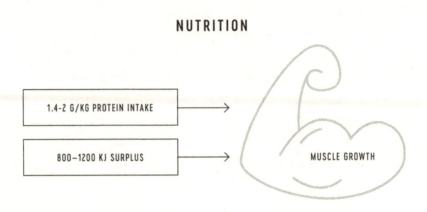

Taking in excess kilojoules so protein is spared for muscle growth is essential for muscle gain. This is where carbohydrate becomes very important. The carbohydrate provides the energy, leaving the protein for muscle growth and repair. Consuming protein during recovery after exercise is important to stimulate muscle growth – around 20 grams is sufficient for most people in recovery food and drinks. See chapter 13, 'Strategies for a Speedy Recovery' (page 139) for more information about this.

PROTEIN POWDERS

Milk protein has been shown to be a superior protein for muscle resynthesis and recovery. It is the base of many commercial protein powders. Protein powders are usually made by filtering milk powder to extract out the desired component, the whey protein. Whey protein isolate has the most protein, while whey protein concentrate has protein together with some carbohydrate.

If you are looking for higher protein, then choose a powder with more protein isolate – these products will be more expensive. A powder with some whey protein concentrate will generally provide sufficient protein along with a small amount of carbohydrate, which can be beneficial for recovery. It may also have a slightly creamier taste.

There are also non-dairy alternatives available, such as pea protein, rice and soy protein. The dairy-based protein powders are very low in lactose, so can still be used by most people with a lactose intolerance.

Protein powders often have suggested serving sizes to provide 30 grams or more of protein per serve. In most cases, this is more than you require. Refer back to your individual protein requirements to determine how much you will need.

Protein powders can be convenient, because they don't require refrigeration like many protein-containing foods do; however, there are plenty of foods that can provide sufficient protein. Check where the products are manufactured. In Australia, manufacturing of protein powders comes under food law, governed by Food Standards Australia New Zealand (FSANZ). I only recommend Australian-manufactured protein powders that are sold in stores, as I am more confident that they have been manufactured under the FSANZ and Good Manufacturing Practice (GMP) standards for Australia.

When working with athletes who will be drug tested, I choose a product with independent third-party testing for substances banned under the Australian Sports Anti-Doping Authority (ASADA) and the World Anti-Doping Authority (WADA). This gives me greater reassurance, although it's still not a 100 per cent guarantee that the product will be free of banned substances. This is important for drug-tested athletes, as if the supplement contains a banned substance it could result in a positive drug test and, subsequently, a ban. The responsibility lies with the athlete, not the supplement company.

GETTING YOUR PROTEIN FROM FOOD

I take a food-first approach to protein intake. Nourishing food choices will contain amino acids (some will contain all nine essential amino acids), together with other valuable nutrients such as antioxidants, vitamins and minerals for cell repair. Protein powders can be used in addition to a balanced diet, but they are not essential. There are plenty of foods containing protein.

PROTEIN CONTENT OF SOME FOODS	
FOOD	PROTEIN CONTENT (GRAMS)
Chicken (100 g)	~30
Beef (100 g)	~28
Fish (100 g)	~25
Yoghurt (100 g)	10
Cheese (20 g, 1 slice)	5
Milk (250 ml, 1 cup)	12
Egg (1 medium)	7
Legumes such as chickpeas, kidney beans (1 cup)	15
Almonds (30 g)	6
Pepitas (30 g)	7
Edamame beans (½ cup)	9
Tofu (100 g)	8

Grains also contain protein, just to a lesser extent. Nonetheless, they do contribute to overall protein intake as they make up a considerable amount of most people's diets. For example:

- » quinoa, 100 grams (½ cup) – 4 grams
- » brown rice, 110 grams (½ cup) – 3 grams
- » pasta, white, 45 grams (½ cup) – 4 grams

Quinoa also contains all the essential amino acids, making it a popular grain protein source.

Eggs are a convenient and easy-to-prepare protein food. The National Heart Foundation of Australia says that it is healthy to eat up to one egg per day, and maybe more for some people. Eggs do contain a small amount of cholesterol, but this is insignificant to total cholesterol levels. What is more important in managing cholesterol levels and risk factors for heart disease is the amount and source of saturated fat and trans fat we eat. An egg contains around 5 grams of total fat, 1.5 grams of which are saturated, which is very little. The rest is unsaturated fat, which is good for our heart and cholesterol levels.

The yolk is rich in iron, selenium, iodine, B-group vitamins, and fat-soluble vitamins A, D and E. Very few foods contain vitamin D, so this is a great benefit. It also contains lutein and zeaxanthin, both carotenoids (compounds that give the yellow colour), which are needed for eye health.

> ### MYTH: EGGS WILL INCREASE YOUR CHOLESTEROL LEVEL
>
> This is a myth: eggs will not increase your cholesterol level (when eating 1–2 a day). Many people believe the nutrient-packed yolk should be avoided due to the cholesterol it contains. What a waste! I think the white and yolk are best eaten together, working in harmony with important nutrient interactions. Let's put a stop to the egg white omelette fad, I say.

Some high-protein-containing foods such as some red meats, and poultry with the skin on, can contain significant amounts of saturated fat. This saturated fat can be kept to a minimum by looking for lean choices and removing the skin from poultry. Chapter 4 will look more closely at our fat requirements.

CHAPTER 4
Fat: The Good, the Bad and the Ugly

The traditional low-fat-everything message, which is commonly pitched at athletes in particular, seems to be changing. We now understand that it is good to eat some fats – but which types, and how much should we have?

TYPES OF FAT

Saturated fat is mainly found in animal products such as meat and dairy, and a few plant sources, such as palm and coconut oil. Saturated fat is also found in lots of processed foods, including biscuits, cakes and pastries. Palm oil is often referred to simply as vegetable oil on food package ingredient listings. It is cheap, 50 per cent saturated fat, and highly processed. When used in baked goods it gives a texture similar to that produced by the inclusion of butter, at a fraction of the price. Avoid it.

Saturated fats have always been painted as evil, but are they really that bad? When they are eaten in highly processed foods they can have adverse effects on your health, so are best kept to a minimum. However, more recent research indicates that saturated fat combined with other nutrients such as protein and minerals (e.g. calcium), for example in dairy foods, may act in a different way to saturated fat consumed in isolation, and may not increase your cholesterol level. So maybe having full-cream milk on your cereal isn't so bad. More research is needed in this area to further understand the effects.

The aim is to keep our bad cholesterol (LDL) levels down and our good cholesterol (HDL) up. In general, total cholesterol levels should be less than 5.5 mmol/litre, and the ratio of good to bad cholesterol is also important. If you have other heart-health risk factors, your recommended levels may be less than 4.5 mmol/litre. This would be something to discuss with your doctor.

It is important to remember that you don't have to be overweight to have high cholesterol. Cholesterol is influenced by a combination of factors, such as what you eat, hereditary factors (family history) and exercise. Even if you exercise regularly and are a healthy weight, you may still have high cholesterol. I have worked with elite athletes in their twenties who are very fit, eat a nutritious diet and still have elevated cholesterol levels. It is important to focus on what foods can be eaten to help reduce cholesterol levels.

While saturated fats have only single-bond joins between carbon molecules, polyunsaturated fats have more than one double bond, and monounsaturated fats have one double bond. Both poly- and monounsaturated fats are referred to as unsaturated fats due to their chemical structure.

Most fats and oils are a combination of saturated, poly- and monounsaturated fat. Polyunsaturated fats provide omega 3 and omega 6 fatty acids, which your body cannot produce, so are essential. Polyunsaturated fats are best obtained from eating wholefood sources such as fish, seeds (such as flaxseeds, sunflower seeds, chia seeds) and nuts (such as walnuts or brazil nuts), as these fats are less stable when processed into cooking oil, and oxidise more readily.

Monounsaturated fats are commonly found in plant foods such as avocado, almonds, cashews and peanuts, and cooking oils such as olive, peanut, canola, rice bran, sunflower and sesame oil.

CHOOSING YOUR OIL

It is important to choose oils that are stable. Oxidative stability, rather than smoke point, is the most important predictor of an oil's stability. Stable oils are naturally produced (unrefined), and contain antioxidants, less polyunsaturated fats and more monounsaturated fats to keep the oil stable when heated. This will minimise harmful polar compounds forming. Polar compounds are free fatty acids and free radicals formed when an oil is exposed to heat. These cannot be digested, and have been shown to be harmful to health. Commercial establishments that use oil for frying are supposed to check the oil for polar compound levels and discard the oil when it reaches a certain polar compound level.

EXTRA VIRGIN OLIVE OIL

The best oil to use for any cooking is extra virgin olive oil (EVOO). Australian EVOO is generally good quality. Olive oil (not EVOO) has been refined, generally using heat and possibly chemicals. EVOO is cold-pressed oil made from fresh olives. EVOO contains a large percentage of monounsaturated fat and has less polyunsaturated fat. It contains antioxidants, and is very stable for all home cooking. Many people incorrectly believe it is not suitable for cooking. Other oils, such as canola oil, will develop polar compounds at a lower temperature than EVOO will. Oil deteriorates with time, so use fresh oil – this is another good reason to buy local produce.

Choose EVOO to splash over your salad and vegetables, to cook your roast, to barbecue – for any cooking at all. It will increase absorption of vitamins, carotenoids (vitamin A) and glucosinolates found in broccoli, cauliflower, kale and cabbage. Adding EVOO may also increase the amount of salad and vegetables you eat, as it makes them more appealing, shiny, moist and tasty. That has to be good for your health!

Inflammation can hit so many of us, particularly the very active, due to overuse of joints and muscles. Joint pain such as arthritis affects around 15 per cent of the Australian population. Studies have suggested that daily consumption of around 50 millilitres (2½ tablespoons) of EVOO per day provides approximately 10 millilitres of oleocanthal, a phenolic compound that seems to have an effect similar to a low dose of ibuprofen. Oleocanthal is found only in EVOO. I encourage athletes not to be scared to use oil.

COCONUT OIL

Coconut oil is around 90 per cent saturated fat, which makes it very stable for cooking. It contains a fatty acid called lauric acid that may increase the good cholesterol, HDL, although it has also been shown to increase the bad cholesterol, LDL. Lauric acid is a medium-chain fatty acid. Short-chain and medium-chain fats are usually absorbed easily, but lauric acid acts like a long-chain fat and travels in the bloodstream to the liver. As it travels, it may be deposited in arteries, increasing LDL cholesterol levels. I suggest using coconut oil sparingly, for its flavour rather than for health benefits. You could always mix some EVOO with coconut oil for health and taste combined.

ENERGY CONTENT OF FATS

All fats contain the same kilojoule (energy) value – 37 kilojoules per gram, the highest of all the macronutrients. This may be a factor to consider if you want to reduce total body weight by reducing total kilojoule intake. However, fat does provide a degree of satiety (feeling of fullness), so it should not be reduced too severely. The type of fat eaten is the most important factor to consider for health.

For people with large energy requirements, such as endurance athletes or growing teenagers, the energy density of fat helps bump up the kilojoules, meaning less volume of food needs to be eaten. I would encourage a young, growing footballer to be more liberal with the higher, good-quality fat choices.

It is important to minimise foods that are sources of poor-quality fats (e.g. saturated fats in processed foods, old oils, trans fats), even if a higher kilojoule intake is required, as these may still be detrimental to health.

FAT AND SATIETY

Fat takes time to digest, therefore it keeps you feeling full. Fat in food influences the hormone leptin, which helps control your hunger signals, telling you when you have had enough to eat. A high-carbohydrate food such as toast, topped with a food containing fat, such as avocado or cheese, for example, will have a greater satiety effect. When weight management is a consideration, working out how much fat to eat is a balancing act. You want enough fat to help fill you up for longer, but not too much, to avoid having excessive kilojoules, as fat is very energy dense.

FAT AND GI

Fat lowers the glycaemic index (GI) of carbohydrate-rich foods when they are eaten together, thus reducing the speed at which a carbohydrate is digested and the glucose enters the bloodstream. That doesn't mean you should go straight to the fish and chip shop, however. It is important to choose quality oils to cook your food in, and these are not generally used in a deep fryer. And remember, too much fat can make you feel sluggish, as it takes longer to digest.

I find balancing fat and carbohydrate important for people who have type 2 diabetes. They need carbohydrate to fuel them, but too much will raise their blood sugar (glucose) levels. Combing carbohydrate-containing foods with those that contain healthy fats can help balance blood glucose levels. Eating foods such as avocado, extra virgin olive oil (EVOO), cheese or a nut spread on a sandwich, nuts or yoghurt with fruit, and choosing a nut bar over a cereal muesli bar are all suitable combinations.

TIPS FOR ADDING HEALTHY FATS INTO YOUR DAY

- » Have a handful of nuts daily for a snack, or include them in a stir-fry or on your breakfast.
- » Drizzle EVOO onto your salads and vegetables with dinner.
- » Brush bread with EVOO instead of butter or margarine.
- » Eat oily fish such as salmon, sardines, mackerel or tuna regularly.
- » Add chia seeds into a smoothie or cake.
- » Bake with EVOO instead of butter.
- » Enjoy avocado as a snack, or smashed on toast for breakfast. Alternatively, spread it onto crackers and top with tomato.
- » Always eat the yolk of the egg as well as the white (the yolk has the fat, minerals and vitamins).
- » Eat lean red and white meat (even lean meat contains around 10 per cent fat).
- » Use 100 per cent nut spread on toast.
- » Drink and eat reduced-fat or full-cream dairy products instead of skim (no fat).
- » Have a slice of cheese for a snack.
- » Add EVOO to mashed potatoes.
- » Stir EVOO through pasta.
- » Add seeds to cereal or smoothies.

CHAPTER 5
Fluid and Hydration

It is generally recommended that we drink eight glasses of water per day. This is a reasonable recommendation, and will be suitable for most of us, however the science doesn't really back this up. We all have different fluid needs, which change depending on body weight, climate, sweat rate, activity level, medical situation and age. So how can you work out what, when and how much to drink to ensure you are well hydrated?

Water is the best drink most of the time, for most people. We are lucky to have a safe water supply in most parts of Australia. Simply turning on the tap is the quickest, most economical and most environmentally sound way of getting water. But even though water is the best drink most of the time, sometimes we would benefit from having more than just water.

DEHYDRATION

Our body is made up of around 60–70 per cent water by weight. Therefore, we need plenty of fluid. Dehydration occurs when the body loses more fluid than it takes in, and the resulting imbalance disrupts the usual levels of electrolytes (salts) and glucose in the blood. There are varying degrees of dehydration, and even a 2 per cent loss of body fluid can have negative effects, such as:

» reduced concentration and decision-making skills
» increased perception of effort during physical activity
(it will feel harder than usual)

- » feeling overheated
- » feeling tired and lethargic
- » headaches
- » overeating, due to confusion between hunger and thirst.

Overall, dehydration can have a negative effect on both your sporting and everyday performance.

On the flip side, we don't want to drink too much water, as this can leave us feeling bloated or weighed down. When I am working with athletes, particularly footballers, we want to hydrate them well, while still ensuring that they feel light and fast.

ARE YOU DEHYDRATED? HOW CAN YOU TELL?

Here are some signs to help identify dehydration:

- » **Urine:** Take a peek in the toilet bowl – what colour do you see? Your urine should be the colour of pale straw, although medications and some supplements can influence the colour. If it is dark yellow, this is an indicator that you need a drink, and are already somewhat dehydrated. This will often occur overnight, with dark urine resulting in the morning. To help reduce this, particularly if you are planning to exercise early in the morning, check your urine colour early in the evening. If it's dark, increase your fluid intake until your urine becomes fairly clear. Try not to drink so much that you will wake to go to the toilet more than once throughout the night, though, as sleep is vital for good health and recovery.

    If your urine is as clear as water, and you are going to the toilet as frequently as you are drinking, back off with the fluid and/or change fluids to one containing electrolytes (see oral rehydration fluids and sports drinks on page 74).

    It is also important to monitor frequency of urination. You should be passing urine at least every 3–4 hours.

- » **Thirst:** Thirst is another guide to help prevent dehydration. When you feel thirsty, your body is reminding you to have a drink. When exercising or in extreme heat, however, this mechanism is less reliable than usual. You are already partly dehydrated when you become thirsty, so ensure you are well hydrated before commencing exercise, and continue to top up regularly.
- » **Heat:** Are you starting to feel overheated when exercising? This may be a sign of dehydration and not being able to adequately cool the body through evaporation of fluid. Also think about the temperature of the training environment and your activity level. On warm days, have more fluid before, during and after activity.
- » **Tired:** If you are feeling tired and yawning, you might need to increase your water intake.
- » **Headaches:** When you are dehydrated you can suffer from headaches. Use the urine colour indicator and see if trying for straw-coloured urine helps relieve the headaches. See a doctor if headaches persist.
- » **Constipation:** Your bowels need fluid to keep stools soft. If you are suffering from constipation, lack of fluid could be a contributing factor.

Once your body is dehydrated it becomes harder to rehydrate, as gastric emptying of fluid can be delayed. As a result, you may start to feel bloated and will rehydrate more slowly. If you feel uncomfortable with fluid in your stomach while exercising, you can practise hydrating during activity, starting with small amounts and building up gradually to what you can tolerate.

Keeping hydrated doesn't mean downing so much water you are running to the toilet constantly. You need a balance of water and electrolytes, and that balance is individual. Let's take a look at how to achieve this balance.

WHAT IS YOUR SWEAT RATE?

Your sweat rate is a measure of how much fluid you lose through sweat during an exercise session or given period of time. You can determine a rough guide by following these steps during a session.

1. Weigh yourself pre- and post-exercise, with minimal clothing on – only underwear is best. (If you leave sweaty clothing on to weigh yourself, you will be weighing the sweat, which is actually lost fluid.) The change in body weight indicates your fluid (sweat) loss.
2. Record the start and finish time of the exercise session.
3. Measure the volume of fluid you drank during the session.
4. The fluid lost (weight change) + fluid drunk = fluid loss.

   This figure, along with the duration of the session, will indicate your sweat rate.

   Fluid loss (in ml) divided by duration of session (minutes) = fluid loss (in ml per minute)

   Fluid loss (in ml per minute) × 60 minutes = fluid loss/hour

   For example, if you exercised for 45 minutes, lost 1 kg and drank 500 ml then your rate = 1500 ml ÷ 45 minutes = 33.3. Multiply this by 45 minutes = 2000 ml per hour.

You can make the sweat loss calculation more accurate by also measuring the volume of urine expelled during the exercise session. Add the volume of urine to the fluid loss figure. An accredited sports dietitian can take you through a sweat-testing session. They may also use sweat patches and measure the sodium level of your sweat to determine whether you are a salty sweater.

> Knowing your fluid loss can guide you in how much you need to drink during exercise. You are not expected to replace all fluid, and certainly don't want to take in more than you lose. Remember that climate and intensity of session will result in a different sweat rate each time.

HOW MUCH SHOULD I DRINK?

It is difficult to give a population-based guide to how much fluid you should drink, given all the influencing factors and differences between individuals. As mentioned earlier, the rough guide of eight glasses a day seems to have stuck. Another measure used is 35 millilitres per kilogram of body weight. Roughly measure how much fluid you currently drink to give yourself a starting point. You can then increase or decrease this according to the signs of dehydration and your sweat rate, depending on conditions As a rough guide, you should be drinking at a rate 125–250 millilitres per 20 minutes of intense exercise. Note how you feel, and avoid drinking more rapidly than fluid can be absorbed, which can leave you feeling bloated. The stomach can absorb around 1 litre per hour. Sweat rates can be this or more, particularly in hot environments.

Remember to drink even if it is cool weather, and when swimming. I have worked with swimmers who neglect their hydration. You still sweat while swimming, you just don't notice it – indoor pools can be very warm, and your body will sweat to try and keep cool.

GETTING THE BALANCE OF FLUID RIGHT

If you are off for a run, in the middle of a match, in an exam at school or a meeting at work, the last thing you want to do is stop to go to the toilet. Then-captain of the Australian cricket team, Ricky Ponting, once reminded me that you can't run off the field for a toilet break, so my pushing of hydration had him 'busting' at times. Getting the balance of fluid volume and electrolyte concentration for retention is essential.

If you are urinating as often as you are drinking water, you can reduce how much water you are having. If you still feel thirsty, consider varying the fluid. Include some fluids that contain electrolytes, such as milk, sports drinks, oral rehydration fluids, milk alternatives (e.g. soy milk), drinking yoghurt, fruit juice (small volumes) or soup.

Healthy kidneys do a great job of balancing how much fluid to retain and filter out along with electrolytes. In general, water will suffice as fluid and food for our electrolytes. Listen to your body and see what it is telling you: thirst, urine volume and colour, energy levels – these signs of dehydration will help you know what approach to take and when. I know when I travel to a hot, humid country I need to take some oral rehydration sachets with me to help replace electrolytes. I sweat much more in these conditions, losing more electrolytes than normal, and if I just drink water I continue to feel thirsty and dehydrated.

Drinking too much water can cause a condition known as hyponatremia. This is rare, and is usually seen in events more than 4 hours long, during which a competitor has drunk too much water and not eaten. (This might occur for example in very humid conditions, where your sweat rate may drop due to evaporation of fluid from the skin being limited as a result of the humidity. If it is a hot and humid climate, you may need to look at other cooling methods in addition to drinking, and use electrolyte-containing fluids. It can also occur in low-intensity exercise if more fluid is drunk than lost. At low intensity, thirst is a good indicator of fluid needs.) When too much water is taken in without enough electrolytes or salts, the body's blood can become too low in sodium. The body then starts to move water out of the blood and into other parts of the body, like the brain, causing confusion. Do not drink more than you sweat out, and if exercising for long periods, eat to provide carbohydrate and electrolytes. Food like fruit contains the electrolyte potassium; bread, crackers and cheese contain salt (sodium); and spreads such as peanut butter and Vegemite also contain salt.

WHAT ARE ELECTROLYTES?

Electrolytes are substances that conduct electrical impulses around our body. Their concentration is tightly controlled in our blood and cells. Electrolytes can be found in food and fluids. The electrolytes contained in sports and oral rehydrating drinks are mostly sodium and potassium, and these drinks can also include minerals such as magnesium, iron and calcium. Sodium and potassium are responsible for maintaining the balance of fluid inside and outside of the cells.

HOW DO I KNOW IF I NEED ELECTROLYTE REPLACEMENT?

How salty your sweat is will affect the quantity of electrolytes you need to replace, in addition to water, in order to maintain optimal hydration. If you leave salt marks on your cap and T-shirt after exercise, your sweat tastes salty (everyone's does, but some people's sweat is stronger than others'), and you can't seem to rehydrate well with just water after exercise, you may need to look at extra electrolyte replacement. In some elite sports, sweat testing may be performed (see page 66). This can help work out more precisely what sort of fluid will best rehydrate an individual. The more concentrated the sweat electrolyte level, the more electrolytes the person will need to take in.

A salty sweater who only drinks water when trying to rehydrate will find that their body doesn't retain the water efficiently, as it needs to balance the concentration of bodily fluids with electrolytes. Excess water will pass out as urine, even though they are not yet hydrated.

The intensity of exercise, duration and climate will also make a difference to what you need to drink, as these affect the quantity of sweat lost. It is the combination of quantity and electrolyte concentration of sweat that needs to be considered in determining the amount and type of food and fluid needed to maximise hydration.

For many of us, obtaining electrolytes from our food and drinking water is sufficient to maintain hydration status, particularly at rest. It is when we become active, particularly at high intensity, that the other factors come into play.

KEEPING ADAM GILCHRIST HYDRATED

Australian cricketer Adam Gilchrist would wicket keep and then be opening batsman in a one-day game. It was a challenge to keep him well hydrated for optimal concentration in hot conditions over long periods.

This is what I recommended for Adam in order to maintain a balance of fluid and electrolytes:

- an electrolyte oral rehydration fluid the evening before a match (~600 ml)
- going to bed with straw-coloured urine
- sipping on water in the morning, and adding milk to breakfast (e.g. in cereal), more oral rehydration fluid (~600 ml) throughout the morning and at the ground. More water if desired.
- some sports drink during play to top him up with carbohydrates if out batting or fielding for some hours and not eating much. If eating, then oral rehydration fluid and water should keep his hydration status and energy levels up. Foods such as soup, yoghurt, fruit or a smoothie would be suitable foods to eat at breaks, as these contribute to fluid, fuel (e.g. carbohydrate) and electrolytes.

He could also add oral rehydration fluid tablets or a powder to the sports drink if he felt he needed the carbohydrate of the sports drink and the extra electrolytes of the oral rehydration fluid.

When working with the Australian Men's Cricket team during the early 2000s, we did sweat testing during a training session in Brisbane. The testing showed that some players had a high sweat volume, while others a smaller volume, but their sweat was saltier. This was of particular importance for those players who were going to bowl for long periods in hot conditions.

We also collected urine samples from the players first thing in the morning and then throughout the day of a test match to check for hydration changes. (Glenn McGrath took great delight in bringing his morning urine sample to breakfast and asking if I would like some apple juice.) The aim was to keep the urine the colour of straw throughout the day's play. Nowadays we have urine-specific gravity testing machines that measure hydration status with just a drop of urine, which the athlete can measure themselves – no more breakfast samples for me! But for most of us, checking our urine colour by peeking in the toilet is reasonably accurate.

Although sometimes we need more than just water alone, plain water is the main fluid, and some of us would benefit from having a little more.

TIPS FOR BOOSTING YOUR WATER INTAKE

- **Make water your preferred drink:** It's good for your teeth, doesn't contain sugar, is readily accessible, cheap and your body likes it.
    - Choose a nice glass.
    - Get the temperature right – do you prefer hot, cold or room temperature?
    - Have it in an easy to reach place, such as on your desk, in a jug on the bench, in the fridge, or on the table with your meal.
- **Flavour water with fruit:** Lemon, lime or orange slices put into the water work well, but only include these in the glass of water that you are about to drink. Acid from the fruit, particularly lemon, can eat away at enamel on your teeth, so don't add it to water you will sip on continuously throughout the day.
- **Drink carbonated waters:** Carbonated waters such as mineral water or soda water can make up part of your water intake. Remember that they contain sodium, varying from very little (supermarket brands) to higher (those from natural springs). Just be aware that the carbonation could increase reflux or bloating from the gas, and these are more acidic than water, so look after your tooth enamel.

WHAT OTHER FLUIDS CAN I DRINK?

- » **Tea:** Cups of tea count as fluid. The weaker the tea, the less caffeine, and there are also a wide variety of herbal teas available. Some research suggests that around three cups of black tea per day provides enough of the amino acid L-theanine to improve concentration.
- » **Coffee:** A standard cup of coffee will still give a positive water balance, even allowing for the diuretic effect of caffeine. Limit quantities and watch the strength. Sometimes you can use caffeine to give you an extra boost in sport. Determine suitable levels for you that won't interfere with sleep or performance.
- » **Milk:** Cow's milk contains the electrolytes sodium, potassium, calcium and phosphorus, which all help with hydration. It also provides calcium for nerve impulse conduction, bone and tooth strength, protein and carbohydrate – perfect for a pre- or post-exercise food and fluid. When I am very thirsty I often crave milk. In fact, milk has similar electrolyte levels to, and greater quantities of potassium than, many sports drinks. Almond milk and other milk alternatives still provide fluid, but with fewer electrolytes and less protein.
- » **Soup or broth:** Soups or broths will provide electrolytes such as sodium (salt), which is particularly beneficial for those active, salty sweaters who need extra sodium together with fluid. For less salty sweaters, keep the salt level moderate and enjoy the fluid. Soup has the added bonus of vegetables for nutrients, protein (if adding meat or legumes) for recovery and carbohydrate (if adding rice, pasta, potatoes, etc.). Soup makes a great healthy snack or meal.
- » **Yoghurt:** A large percentage of yoghurt is water. You can also add water to yoghurt, making it into a milk drink, or buy fermented milk drinks (probiotic milks) – think kefir and Filmjölk. However, yoghurt made from cow's milk contains electrolytes, protein and calcium.
- » **Fruit juice:** Fruit juice contains plenty of vitamins, but with around 10 per cent sugar (the same sugar percentage as soft drink), it's only suitable if you need to replace large amounts of carbohydrate, and is also quite acidic, which your tooth enamel does not like. Fruit juice does contain the electrolyte potassium, but the high

sugar concentration can slow the uptake of water from the gut. Small amounts are okay, but I do not recommend fruit juice as your main fluid intake.

» **Coconut water:** Contrary to popular belief, coconut water is not a miracle hydrating fluid. It is similar in composition to water, and contains minimal electrolytes. If you are looking for some flavour and like the taste, it will add to your fluid intake.

» **Oral rehydration fluids:** Originally designed to rehydrate after illness, such as gastroenteritis or diarrhoea, these are designed specifically to rehydrate you when you have lost large amounts of electrolytes and fluid. They are made to the World Health Organization's formula, and are often used in developing countries. Oral rehydration solutions are higher in electrolytes (around 4 × more than sports drinks) and much lower in sugar than traditional sports drinks (~ 2–3 vs. 7–8 per cent).

I find the low sugar content of oral rehydration fluids to be a big advantage, as most of us do not need the sugar found in other beverages. However, they do tend to have an artificial sweetener added to help mask the salty flavour, and if consuming large volumes these sweeteners can sometimes cause gut upset. The electrolytes of an oral rehydration fluid help retain water and replace electrolytes lost through sweat.

They are also useful when travelling, as planes can be dehydrating environments. If you have had too much alcohol, electrolyte-containing drinks will be your friend, as the hangover feeling has a lot to do with dehydration. However, drinking less alcohol is an easier option.

» **Sports drinks:** These are designed for the very active. Containing around 7 per cent carbohydrate or sugar, sports drinks provide energy as well as electrolytes. The sugar and electrolytes speed up the uptake of water, which is important for intense activity lasting longer than 60–90 minutes. However, it is important to consider whether you need this much sugar, or if you could obtain the carbohydrate from food. The flavour of sports drinks usually results in more fluid being drunk, which is important for endurance-type activities or in very hot conditions. An accredited sports dietitian can help you decide whether these are needed, how much and when.

- **Soft drink and energy drinks:** If I had a list of banned foods and fluids, soft drink and energy drinks would be on it. At 10 per cent sugar, it is so easy to drink more than your daily sugar needs from just one can: 8 teaspoons, with no other nutritional value. The sugar and citric acid used to make soft drink also result in a drink with a low pH (meaning they are acidic), which affects our teeth. A pH below 4 can start to dissolve the outer layer of our tooth enamel, increasing the likelihood of tooth decay, and the bacteria in our mouth uses the sugar to produce acid that also dissolves and damages our teeth.

    Soft drink does not provide any electrolytes, and the high sugar level can slow the rate of fluid emptying from the stomach. There is, of course, plenty of water in the soft drink, so it does provide fluid, but it's not an option I would recommend. Keep soft drink to a minimum.

- **Alcohol:** I think we all know that alcohol can be dehydrating due to its effects on the hormones that control the kidneys. That is partly what causes the feeling of being hungover. Although a drink or two will not cause dehydration, alcohol is not the best choice to aid hydration, particularly after exercise, when your body is trying to repair. Alcohol causes blood vessel dilation, which could exacerbate any bleeding from bruising. The advice is to rehydrate before drinking alcohol, and to choose the lowest percentage alcohol-containing drinks, such as light beer. See page 80 for more information about its dehydrating effect.

Athletes I work with drink varying combinations of fluids to keep hydrated, but mostly water. Post-game, some of the Hawthorn players like to drink chocolate-flavoured milk. As soon as they leave the field I give them protein milk drinks to provide protein, carbohydrate, water and electrolytes, plus extra protein and chocolate flavour, if a protein powder is added.

When it comes to hydration in sport, sponsorship issues can be a headache. When working with the Australian Men's Cricket team, the ground was sponsored by one sports drink company, and the team by another. We had to bring in our own, non-branded fridges, as we were not allowed to have rival sports drinks, or bottled water, in the ground's fridges, which had opposition sponsorship on them.

DOES DEHYDRATION CAUSE CRAMPING?

If you have experienced a cramp during exercise you'll know how debilitating it can be. These cramps are often referred to as Exercise-Associated Muscle Cramps (EAMC).

There are a number of theories to explain what causes cramping during exercise, with the most likely being fatigue in the exercising muscle. This is why cramps most commonly occur in the muscle groups directly involved in the exercise.

We often talk about inadequate electrolyte levels (e.g. potassium, magnesium or calcium) being the cause for cramps, but the research is not convincing. Dehydration has also been claimed to be the cause of cramps, but again, the research doesn't support this. However, being well hydrated can help prevent cramps, as dehydration may contribute to fatigue of the muscle, which can increase the risk of cramping. Just as dehydration can have an indirect effect on cramping, so too can inadequate fuel – again because the muscle may prematurely fatigue and then cramp.

In recent years, pickle juice has been used to help stop cramping. The pickle juice, which is a salty, acidic solution, is thought to stop the electrical signal that causes electrically induced muscle cramps. More research is needed to understand the exact mechanism, but swallowing around 30–60 millilitres, or swirling it in the mouth, can alleviate cramping in around a minute. This might be something to consider if cramping is an issue, but sufficient training and conditioning of muscles to prevent fatigue is the best way to alleviate cramps.

CHAPTER 6
Is Alcohol Allowed?

Many people enjoy an alcoholic drink with few adverse effects to their health. It is worthwhile knowing the safe drinking limits set by the National Health and Medical Research Council (NH&MRC), as a substantial number of people do drink more, and suffer adverse effects to their health and their lives. Drinking alcohol can also have an adverse effect on performance, which is important to consider if striving for peak performance.

The NH&MRC 2009 guidelines (currently under review) recommend:

- » For healthy men and women, having no more than two standard drinks on any day reduces the lifetime risk of harm from alcohol-related disease or injury.
- » Every drink above this level continues to increase the lifetime risk of both disease and injury.
- » Drinking less frequently over a lifetime (e.g. drinking weekly, rather than daily), and drinking less on each drinking occasion, reduces the lifetime risk of alcohol-related harm.

There are also guidelines around teenage drinking, and during pregnancy and lactation.

A standard drink is 10 grams of alcohol, which equates to:

- » 100 millilitres of wine
- » 250 millilitres of full-strength beer
- » 30 millilitres of a spirit.

Restaurants tend to pour 150-millilitre glasses of wine, which equates to 1.5 standard drinks, and a stubby of beer is 375 millilitres, which is 1.4 standard drinks.

There is always talk about the antioxidants in red wine and the benefits to heart health from the polyphenols and flavonoids it contains, such as resveratrol. Wine does contain some antioxidants, but so do a whole range of foods. By all means enjoy a glass of wine if that suits your health, but don't take up drinking for health benefits – try eating a bunch of red grapes instead.

It is worth knowing a little about the effects alcohol has on the body. Alcohol is absorbed quickly, not requiring digestion, and can reach the brain in less than one minute if drunk on an empty stomach. It passes from the gut to the bloodstream and then straight to the brain – in other words, it gets an express pass. Alcohol travels to all parts of the body, especially the brain, kidneys and liver.

Once absorbed, the alcohol travels in the blood to the liver, where the enzyme alcohol dehydrogenase starts to break it down. There are numerous breakdown reactions that occur from then on, interfering with the liver's usual function. The liver usually prefers to break down fatty acids (fat) for a lot of our fuel source, together with carbohydrate. Metabolising the alcohol reduces or blocks these pathways, meaning fatty acids accumulate, rather than being broken down. An accumulation of fat in the liver can be observed after only a single night of heavy drinking. Excessive alcohol intake over time can mean that the storage of fatty acids results in a 'fatty' liver. You can have a blood test that measures liver function, and this is worth doing if you think this might be a concern. Your liver is your very own chemical processing plant, constantly making and breaking things down. Look after it.

The liver can only break down about one standard drink per hour. You cannot speed this process up with coffee, cold showers or any other methods you might think up. It simply takes time, and the amount of time it takes depends on our genetically determined liver enzyme function.

ALCOHOL CONTRIBUTES TO WEIGHT GAIN

Perhaps it is the off season, the end of the week, or you might be celebrating a win, or a personal best, and think you might have an alcoholic beverage or two. If body fat levels are an important consideration, then think about how much alcohol you are planning to have. It is the alcohol in the drink that contributes to body fat gain, rather than the carbohydrate. The energy or kilojoule value of alcohol is far greater than that of carbohydrate:

- » alcohol = 27 kilojoules per gram
- » carbohydrate = 16 kilojoules per gram
- » fat = 39 kilojoules per gram
- » protein = 17 kilojoules per gram.

Because the body must first break down the alcohol, this means fat is stored rather than being broken down. When drinking, we are also sometimes less selective in our food choices, opting for greasy takeaway instead of healthier choices. The combination of alcohol and less nutritious food is a double whammy.

LOW-CARB BEERS

There is a misconception that low-carbohydrate beers are better than standard beers – this is just clever marketing. Although the carbohydrate content is slightly less, it's not significantly so in most cases. In addition, some people end up drinking more, thinking it is healthier.

Carbohydrate content is far more significant in soft drink than in beer:

- » 375 ml can of soft drink = 40 g of carbohydrate   0% alcohol
- » 375 ml full-strength beer = ~10 g of carbohydrate   4.8% alcohol
- » 375ml low-carb beer = ~3.5 g of carbohydrate   4.8% alcohol

The 7-gram difference in carbohydrate between the beers is negligible, especially considering that many of us require 310 grams or more of carbohydrate per day (based on an average daily kilojoule value of 8700 kJ/day). If you are having numerous beers, that 'saving' might add up, but the real issue is that the alcohol content is the same. You are better off choosing a low-alcohol drink (around 2.7 per cent alcohol) instead, or, better still, keeping your number of alcoholic drinks down.

ALCOHOL AND DEHYDRATION

Alcohol decreases the body's production of antidiuretic hormone (ADH) in the posterior pituitary gland of your brain, the hormone responsible for reabsorbing water. A reduction causes your kidneys to let go of more water than usual. We usually produce around 60–80 millilitres of urine per hour. Every 10 grams of alcohol can increase this by 120 millilitres per hour. This means the body then loses more water than usual through urination. You will lose more water than the alcoholic drink provides, contributing to dehydration. After exercise, the body changes hormone levels to try and promote rehydration, so the effect of the alcohol on ADH may not be as severe. That does not mean large volumes of alcohol will have no effect. Research has shown that one, and no more than two, beers of mid- to lower alcohol level (~ 3.5 per cent) can contribute to rehydration like a non-alcoholic beverage can. It can also be an important part of the social interaction around exercise. This doesn't suggest you start drinking beer for rehydration, but if you do enjoy one beer after exercise, you can safely do so.

'I will drink more water to counteract the extra loss,' you say. Although this will help, the end result will still be dehydration if you have a big night. Your body will only reabsorb around half of the extra water you drink. That said, you will be better off as a result of having some water. Throw some electrolytes such as an oral rehydration sachet into your water and that will help you retain more fluid.

Milk is also a great choice, providing fluid and electrolytes to help rehydrate you. Kahlua and milk anyone? (Just joking!)

ALCOHOL POST-EXERCISE

If you have been exercising, particularly in a contact sport, it's best to avoid alcohol for at least 24–48 hours afterwards, to aid recovery. Soft-tissue injury management means reducing blood flow to the area in order to contain the injury. Alcohol has the opposite effect – it increases blood flow to the area, which is likely to extend recovery time and exacerbate the injury. It can also increase blood pooling and bruising.

After any exercise session, the aim is to get the body back to a building state (anabolic) rather than breaking down (catabolic). Repairing muscle and muscle gain are often the key goals. If you drink alcohol around this time, you are reducing many of your exercise benefits. Alcohol reduces the levels of the anabolic hormones such as growth hormone and testosterone (which is important in both men and women). Given that growth hormone is produced more during the early parts of your sleep, and alcohol can interfere with your sleep, drinking alcohol can reduce the release of these hormones. (However, one drink is unlikely to have a negative impact and can be enjoyed if desired.)

Glycogen synthesis occurs in the liver. This is particularly important after exercise, to replace the energy used and needed for the next session. When you drink alcohol, the alcohol must first be dealt with, as it is a toxin to the body. While the liver is busy doing this, it is not restoring your glycogen. This delays glycogen synthesis, meaning you may not recover sufficiently before your next exercise session. This is especially important for people who exercise regularly.

GUIDELINES FOR A NIGHT OUT

Enjoying an alcoholic drink can be enjoyable when relaxing with friends or celebrating a win, but remember, it's not compulsory – it is up to you. A fun time can be had both with and without alcohol. The following are some practical suggestions to help you control your intake, rather than letting others dictate it:

1. **Plan:** How many social occasions are you attending this week? Which would you like to have a drink at and which not? Where are you at with training and competition, if that is relevant?

2. **Eat before and/or while you are drinking:** Have something to eat before you start drinking alcohol, or within the couple of hours prior. This can help slow your drinking pace. Food can also slow down the absorption of the alcohol somewhat.
3. **Eat carbohydrate-rich foods after exercise:** It helps replenish muscle fuel stores. Try to eat before you have an alcoholic drink.
4. **Pace yourself:** Space alcoholic drinks with non-alcoholic drinks. Start with a non-alcoholic beverage to quench your thirst. You will drink faster if you are thirsty, particularly after exercise.
5. **Drink slowly:** Sip your drink, and enjoy the taste. Put your glass down between sips.
6. **Volunteer to be designated driver:** If you have made the decision not to drink and are worried that your friends or teammates might pressure you to have a few, let them know that you are driving.
7. **Drink one drink at a time:** Stop people topping up your drink. It makes it hard to track how much you have drunk. (Beware of waiters who may be trying to please you/get you to drink more so you'll buy more.)
8. **Keep yourself busy:** If you are occupied, you tend to drink less. Have a dance, play pool, help cook, move around and talk to others.
9. **Avoid rounds or 'shouts':** Drinking in a 'shout' encourages you to drink at someone else's pace. If you do get stuck in this situation, buy a non-alcoholic drink for yourself when it is your turn, or simply pass.
10. **Rehydrate before you go to bed:** Make sure you drink water, milk or a sports drink before you go to sleep. Have a glass by the bed.

 ## COOKING WITH ALCOHOL

When you cook with alcohol, the alcohol breaks down so it doesn't have the intoxicating effect. Enjoy your wine in a bolognaise, risotto or in a marinade.

CHAPTER 7

Salt

HOW MUCH SALT DO I NEED?

How much salt you require differs depending on a range of factors that influence your salt losses. The National Heart Foundation recommends around 1 teaspoon of salt – 6 grams, or 2300 milligrams of sodium – a day, and around 4 grams for those with high blood pressure. Too much salt can increase the risk of high blood pressure for some, though for those who are less salt sensitive, it may not. Reducing salt intake is generally recommended – heart disease is one of Australia's biggest killers, and high blood pressure is one of the risk factors, which a high salt intake may contribute to.

Having too little salt is not good for your health either. If you have a very restrictive diet with no added salt and minimal processed foods, for example, which generally contain a lot of salt, you may need to add some salt to your diet, particularly if you are sweating significantly.

Our body balances sodium in our blood and cells very carefully. Sodium is used to transmit nerve impulses (such as signals for muscle contraction) and to maintain blood pressure and fluid balance of the body. The body balances fluid coming in and going out, and sodium has a big influence on this. If too much fluid goes out and not enough comes in, we begin to dehydrate. It is your kidneys that do most of the work in balancing sodium and fluid, removing or retaining water to keep the blood concentrations of sodium and other electrolytes correct.

The salt used in home cooking, table salt, is chemically known as sodium chloride. There is salt in many foods we eat daily – for example, breakfast cereal, bread, sauces, condiments, processed meat, cheese, savoury processed snack foods like biscuits, spreads, takeaway food and more. Processed foods give us about 75 per cent of our recommended daily salt, without needing to add any extra at the table.

My mum is a salt lover – sometimes her food looks like it's covered in snow! My kids say, 'Stop, that's enough!', and her excuse is always, 'There isn't much coming out of the shaker,' despite the visible layer all over her food. Thankfully, she eats very few packaged foods that are high in salt. Look at your sodium intake, and remember, it's not just what comes out of the shaker – many foods contain hidden salt. You can wean your taste buds towards desiring less salt.

How much salt do active people need? Most of us have more sodium than we need, so even if we're losing some in sweat, we're still meeting our sodium requirements. People who sweat extreme amounts, work outdoors or in hot environments, or are keen athletes (recreational or professional) may need more salt to account for electrolyte losses.

If excessive sweating occurs, extra sodium can come from salty food and fluids such as oral rehydration fluids and sports drinks. Oral rehydration fluids have much higher sodium levels and less sugar than sports drinks. As the sodium level rises, the taste of the beverage can decline. For active hydration, oral rehydration fluids will be more effective, so it is important to trial these and get used to the taste.

Before long events it can be helpful to eat some foods containing sodium, such as pretzels, Vegemite, cheese, or adding soy sauce or other sauces to food. The salt will increase your thirst, prompting you to drink more, and will help retain the fluid by balancing water and sodium within the body's cells.

When working with athletes, and particularly when I was working with the Australian cricket team, I recommend that players eat some salty foods the night before and the day of matches, as playing in extreme heat for long periods can mean they lose extra sodium in their sweat. I know when I have been in the garden for several hours on a warm day, I become extremely thirsty, and find that just drinking water has me running to the toilet regularly and still feeling thirsty, as my body can't retain the fluid without adequate sodium replacement. I find milk a good solution, as it contains some sodium and other electrolytes to replace losses without having so much that it goes the other way and causes thirst. A glass of an oral rehydration solution also works well for me. Maybe I am a salty sweater.

Are you a salty sweater? Have a look at your cap or T-shirt after sweating. Any white marks? This is sodium that has dried with the sweat, and can be one indicator of losing salt in your sweat. A more scientific method is to conduct a sweat test (see page 66). Sweat is generally between 40 and 80 mmol/litre concentration of sodium, so the results are compared to this range. Sports dietitians are still collecting data about athletes to see what results really mean and whether athletes fit into the average person's range, or if they adapt and lose less sodium in their sweat.

An accredited sports dietitian can conduct a sweat test, and will help you understand the results. You can also conduct a fluid balance study to find out how much fluid you lose per hour. With this information, along with the concentration of your sweat, you can develop a plan around what type of fluid you need, how much, and how much sodium you need to stay hydrated.

It is important to find the balance of salt needed. Too much salt intake will make you thirsty, because the body tries to balance the excess sodium by driving thirst to increase water intake. You will keep feeling thirsty until your body balances its sodium levels.

REDUCING SALT INTAKE

Most of us eat plenty or too much sodium. If you want to reduce your salt intake you may need to retrain your tastebuds and cut back gradually. Flavour your food with herbs and spices (e.g. oregano, basil, paprika, cumin), black pepper, chilli, and mushrooms, which have an earthy, salty taste. Increasing your intake of potassium, found in fruit and vegetables, can also help balance out your sodium levels.

Under the Australia New Zealand Food Standards Code, low-salt foods are those with 120 milligrams or less of sodium per 100 grams. To keep your salt intake in check, look for foods with less than 400 milligrams of sodium per 100 grams.

By monitoring how you feel when exercising (energy levels, dehydration status), your thirst in general, your overall hydration status and knowing risk factors such as your blood pressure and family history of heart disease, you can work out what your salt intake should be.

CHAPTER 8

The Immune System

We all want to boost our immune system. Diet, sleep, rest, relaxation and exercise all have an impact on this. Exercise can be both beneficial and stressful. We have been told exercise is good for our health, and it is. It offers cardiovascular benefits, bone strength, mental health – the list goes on.

Moderate levels of regular exercise (i.e. 1–2 hours of moderate activity) seem to reduce the risk of infection compared to a sedentary lifestyle, but intense exercise (more than 90 minutes at 55–75 per cent aerobic capacity) increases the risk. It puts your body under stress, releasing the stress hormones cortisol and adrenaline, which suppress white blood cell function and therefore the immune system. This leaves you more vulnerable to upper respiratory tract infections like colds and tonsillitis. Having some carbohydrate straight after exercise may help reduce the stress hormone response, bringing levels back to normal more quickly. This is where strategies for recovery food are important (see chapter 13, page 139).

LET'S GET YOUR IMMUNE SYSTEM AT ITS BEST

The immune system is complex. It involves barriers such as the skin, the digestive tract (gut), the nasal passages, the eyes and the respiratory tract. If pathogens are not stopped by these barriers, then other parts of the immune system, namely the lymphatic and blood system, start their work. A healthy diet will help your body be at its best so it can fight off those unwanted pathogens. There isn't one food alone that will do the trick, though – such a complex system requires many nutrients to function.

1. **Healthy gut microbiota:** Having healthy gut bacteria (microbiota) boosts your immune system's defence via the gut by forming a physical barrier to limit the invasion of pathogens through the gut wall. Microbiota can also reduce the number of harmful bacteria and harmful by-products (toxins) they produce. To maximise the immune system we want to introduce good bacteria and ensure that the ones we have flourish. Here are a few tips – refer to chapter 9, 'Maximising Your Gut's Performance' for further details (see page 93).

    a. Eat foods containing good bacteria regularly. These are referred to as probiotics (live microorganisms that, when ingested in adequate amounts, provide a health benefit to the host). Note, a product that claims to contain 'live microorganisms' does not necessarily have a probiotic effect. To be labelled probiotic, the food must contain at least 1 billion live bacteria known to have a health benefit. Yoghurts are a good example, but read the label, and look for the number of colony-forming units per serve, as many yoghurts are low in bacteria numbers.

    Bacteria in fermented milk beverages like probiotic milk Filmjölk, kefir, Yakult and other similar brands have higher bacteria levels, so can be called probiotic drinks. Yoghurt and fermented milk drinks have the added benefit of protein and carbohydrate, making them a good choice for recovery foods.

    Other fermented foods like sauerkraut and pickled vegetables, if unpasteurised or made by you at home, will contain beneficial bacteria and may be worth including in the diet. Unpasteurised products will be found in the refrigerated section of the shop.

    Fermented tea drinks such as kombucha also contain strains of bacteria. They are a tasty drink, and a good alternative to alcoholic drinks and soft drink, as they contain much less sugar. More research needs to be conducted into fermented drinks and foods to understand which bacteria survive the gut, how many are needed for a probiotic benefit, what the individual strains are beneficial for and how these interact with and influence your own gut bacteria.

    b. Eat foods that feed your good gut bacteria. This means foods containing prebiotic fibres like resistant starch. Resistant starch is found in a range of foods, including grains, legumes, bananas, cashew nuts, and cooked cold potatoes and pasta (an added benefit of leftovers).

2. **Protein:** Protein has many functions in the immune system, including making antibodies and forming white blood cells. Making sure there is sufficient protein in your diet will support your immune system.

3. **Vitamins:** We need many vitamins, particularly vitamins A and C, to enable white blood cells and lymphocytes to do their job properly. There is research to support the belief that vitamin C helps reduce the severity and duration of the common cold and flu. Having fruit, and, in particular, raw vegetables such as in salads (as some vitamin C is destroyed upon heating) will boost your vitamin C intake.

Raw red capsicum has more vitamin C than an orange. Strawberries contain about the same amount as an orange, while kiwifruit, broccoli and berries are also all rich sources of vitamin C. Vitamin C is water soluble, meaning it is not stored by the body – excess vitamin C is excreted through your urine. Therefore, it is important to include it regularly in your diet.

4. **Minerals:**

    a. Zinc is crucial for the development and function of the immune system and T cells (a type of white blood cell), which are important in fighting infection. Zinc is also believed to help fight the common cold, although strong, research-based evidence is lacking. Zinc also aids in wound healing. Foods high in zinc include seafood, lamb, beef, whole grains, pepitas and baked beans.

    b. Iron is also important for the immune system. If iron levels in the body are low, such as in people suffering from anaemia, there is an increased risk of infection. If someone is getting sick regularly, it is worth checking their iron levels in case they are low.

    Iron is found in foods such as red and white meat, fish, green leafy vegetables and legumes.

Iron is better absorbed from animal foods in what we call the haem form. In plants, iron is found in non-haem form, and needs a chemical oxidation reaction to change it to the haem form so it can be absorbed. Eating foods rich in vitamin C (ascorbic acid) along with the plant facilitates this reaction, due to the acidic nature of vitamin C. Eating capsicum, tomatoes, beetroot or broccoli with your iron-containing leafy greens and legumes, or eating fruit after a meal to provide vitamin C will help with iron absorption.

When exercising intensely, particularly for endurance events, more iron is needed to replace and make extra red blood cells. During high-altitude competitions or training, your body requires more iron to produce extra red blood cells. This is part of the adaptation to this climate.

5. **Extra virgin olive oil:** Inflammation is part of the immune system's response to injuries and harmful things entering the body. We want to avoid foods that cause extra inflammation, and eat foods that reduce it.

    Trans fats, most commonly found in commercially prepared packaged foods such as pastries, fried foods and biscuits, can increase inflammation in the body, so minimise trans fats in the diet.

    Choosing healthy monounsaturated fats that contain antioxidants, such as extra virgin olive oil, oil in avocados and some of the oil in nuts, is your best choice for minimising inflammation. Cook your vegetables and meats in extra virgin olive oil, and spread avocado or extra virgin olive oil on your bread instead of processed, fatty spreads.

6. **Phytochemicals**: Many of the phytochemicals in fruits and vegetables act as antioxidants, protecting our cells from oxidation, which can produce free radicals and damage cells. Phytochemicals are involved in fighting infection. The recommended two servings of fruit and five of vegetables a day is a good start to having a healthy phytochemical intake for your immune system.

7. **Alcohol:** Avoid binge and excessive alcohol drinking after strenuous exercise and competition, as it suppresses the immune system for some hours.

Try these perfect immune-boosting post-exercise snacks:

» Fresh fruit with yoghurt, sprinkled with cashew nuts and seeds
» A bowl of potato salad with some tuna thrown in, and an extra virgin olive oil and yoghurt dressing
» A smoothie with probiotic milk, banana or berries and chia seeds

WHAT IS IT ABOUT CHICKEN SOUP?

If you have a cold, what better food to have than a bowl of chicken and vegetable soup? The steam helps relieve your blocked nose, and you can add some garlic, ginger and chilli to help too. Including vitamin C–containing vegetables such as cabbage, capsicum, leafy greens and potato will help your immune system. The chicken will provide the protein, zinc and iron you need to help your system fight the infection. If you are not a meat eater you could try adding some legumes instead. Soup seems to be more than just the nutrients it provides – there's also something comforting about the warm liquid when you feel unwell.

CHAPTER 9
Maximising Your Gut's Performance

I often emphasise to athletes just how important gut health is to their overall health and performance. If an athlete's health is not optimal, it's hard for their performance to be. Gut health significantly affects numerous aspects of our overall health, including:

- immune system function
- inflammation
- fatigue
- mood
- depression
- hormone control
- disease risk, e.g. bowel cancer.

When we say 'the gut', we are referring to the gastrointestinal system. This starts at your mouth (oral cavity), and includes the stomach, small and large intestine (also referred to as the small and large bowel) and the organs involved in digestion, finishing at the rectum and anus. That is a significant proportion of the body.

Another important component of the human gut are the more than one trillion bacteria throughout. These make up the gut microbiome, which plays a very important role in one's health. In this section I am going to focus primarily on the influence of the small and large intestines, and how their health affects your overall health and performance.

Gut health issues can be quite distressing. The Gut Foundation of Australia reports that half our population complain of some digestive problem, such as heartburn, diarrhoea, irritable bowel syndrome (IBS), diverticulitis, Crohn's disease and bowel cancer, in any twelve-month period. The rates are increasing, and we know that a healthy diet has positive influence.

You may suffer one or more symptoms such as bloating, abdominal discomfort, excessive flatulence and irregular bowel motions. If you don't, that's great – keep looking after your gut health!

HOW WOULD YOU RATE YOUR BOWEL FORM AND FREQUENCY?

One measure of bowel health is to look at your stool (faeces or poo) form and note its regularity. How often we use our bowels is very individual. Normal stool frequency can be anything from three times a day to once every few days. Not having a daily bowel motion does not mean you are constipated. Constipation is performing a bowel motion less than three times a week, producing hard stool form around a quarter of the time, often requiring medication to assist and without experiencing a feeling of complete emptiness when leaving the toilet. It is more to do with the difficulty of passing the stools than the frequency. It can be very uncomfortable.

Short-term constipation can occur as a result of changes in environment, which is an issue for those who travel regularly, including many athletes I work with. The gut is a creature of habit – it likes routine. When this is disrupted, the usual nerve signals are not sent, so the gut puts everything on hold until it feels comfortable again. This can also happen with unfamiliar toilets, which is something to be aware of. For example, if you are travelling for a competition, you may need to allow time for your gut to 'settle in' to the new surroundings.

Bowels seem to respond to stressful situations in a variety of ways, probably due to the 'gut brain nerve interaction' at work. The gut–brain axis involves two-way communication between the central nervous system (including the brain and spinal cord and nerves, particularly the vagus nerve) in the brain, and the enteric nervous system (the nerves that govern the gut) in the gastrointestinal system. It links the cognitive and emotional centres of the brain with the intestinal functions. Stress activates nerves, which may then affect the gut in different ways, such as by causing diarrhoea, nausea or the feeling of butterflies. Frequent diarrhoea can have a negative impact on hydration, particularly if the feeling of an upset stomach makes it hard to drink to replace the lost fluid.

I once worked with an AFL player who often experienced loose bowels at half time. This may have been due to game nerves, gut–brain association, overstimulation of the vagus nerve in the gut, pain medication taken before a game – there are numerous possibilities. We looked at possible food causes (e.g. lactose, high fibre, caffeine), none of which seemed to be the problem, and settled on a pre-game meal that he felt comfortable with that didn't exacerbate the issue. By making simple changes, we were able to minimise the aggravation.

Bowel habits can also change as a result of hormonal changes, particularly in females, who can sometimes experience a looser bowel at certain times of their menstrual cycle.

The bowel is a muscle, which is stimulated along with other muscles during exercise. This can be annoying if you're out on a long run without a toilet nearby. People who exercise regularly often find that this effect tends to decline over time.

Stool type varies, but in general should be soft and sausage-like in shape most of the time. Dr Ken Heaton from the University of Bristol developed the Bristol stool chart in 1997 to help with diagnosis of digestive problems. An ideal stool is type 3–4 – not too watery and easy to pass. A type 1–2 is likely to be a sign of constipation, and 5–7 possibly diarrhoea. Read the chart to work out where you fit on the scale, remembering that this is only one measure of bowel function.

Whatever your frequency, any major changes in your bowel habits, texture, colour or blood in stools should be discussed with a health professional. Bowel cancer is one of the main cancer-related killers in Australia.

	BRISTOL STOOL CHART
	TYPE 1 Separate hard lumps, like nuts (hard to pass)
	TYPE 2 Sausage-shaped, but lumpy
	TYPE 3 Sausage-shaped, but with cracks on surface
	TYPE 4 Sausage or snake like, smooth and soft
	TYPE 5 Soft blobs with clear-cut edges (easy to pass)
	TYPE 6 Fluffy pieces with ragged edges, mushy
	TYPE 7 Watery, no solid pieces (entirely liquid)

TACKLING THE 'NERVOUS GUT' RESPONSE BEFORE COMPETITION

The way the gut reacts to situations can be debilitating to sporting performance. It's relatively easy to deal with the 'butterflies' you experience due to nerves, but a symptom such as diarrhoea is not only dehydrating, but also very inconvenient! A nervous gut can cause changes in bowel habits ranging from diarrhoea to constipation, bloating and general discomfort. Athletes suffering from irritable bowel syndrome (IBS) can experience particularly severe symptoms.

To resolve issues stemming from a nervous gut, it's important to find strategies that work for you.

» Carbohydrate loading for endurance events might need to be more gradual, starting further ahead of the event and not loading as much the day before.

» Spreading food intake out can help avoid stomach distention and bloating. It is important to consider this if you are trying to carbohydrate load – careful planning may be needed.

» Reducing FODMAP (see page 108) intake before an event (not long-term) can help if you experience symptoms such as bloating, diarrhoea or pain.

» Work out which foods trigger responses for you and avoid eating these on race day.

» Try having some carbohydrate foods before and during the event.

» Keep up hydration to ensure that gastric emptying is not delayed.

> » Seek relaxation strategies and work with a sports psychologist to help reduce the 'nervous gut'. Hypnotism with gut-trained specialists has shown positive results for some people with IBS issues.
>
> The gastrointestinal system is very complex and highly individual, and is an area in which we still have much to learn. Seek advice from a health professional such as an accredited practising dietitian, GP or gastroenterologist. It is also important to listen to how your gut is feeling so you know what works and is normal for you.

DIETARY FIBRE FOR GUT HEALTH

Now that we understand our own bowel habits a little more, we can talk about how diet influences gut health, starting with dietary fibre. Dietary fibre not only provides bulk to stools to keep them moving through the large intestine and to aid defecation (laxation effect), it also helps modulate blood glucose levels and reduce cholesterol. Some fibres also have the capacity to strongly influence your colony of good gut bacteria, therefore affecting both gut health and overall health and wellbeing.

Dietary fibre is found in the parts of plant foods that we cannot digest or absorb. It passes through the stomach and small intestine relatively unchanged, then continues on to the large intestine, where it is partially or fully fermented.

There are different types of dietary fibre, including soluble fibre, insoluble fibre and resistant starch.

» **Soluble fibre:** This is a part of plants, such as pectin, gums, beta-glucan and psyllium, which is found in fruit, vegetables, oats, barley, seed husks, peas, legumes and soy. Soluble fibre may help with maintaining blood glucose levels in the 'healthy' range, and with cholesterol control. It also soaks up fluid to soften stools, which helps prevent constipation.

- **Insoluble fibre:** This comes from the more structural parts of the plant, such as lignin and cellulose. Insoluble fibre provides much of the bulk to your faeces. It is found in wheat, barley, rice and corn bran, seeds, fruit and vegetable skins, and whole grains. Many foods contain both insoluble and soluble fibre.
- **Resistant starch:** This is found in cooked potatoes, pasta and rice that have been left to cool, unripe bananas, lentils, legumes, corn, barley, some whole grains, cashews and dates. It is made up of starch that cannot be digested in the small intestine and so makes its way to the large intestine, where it is consumed by the good bacteria living there. When the bacteria eat resistant starch and other fibres, this is called fermentation. As the good bacteria ferment the resistant starch and other fermentable fibres, they:
    - produce short-chain fatty acids such as butyrate gas, which is healthy for the large intestine and for overall health. Next time someone complains about your gas (flatulence, fart, wind), remind them that it's healthy!
    - provide food for the good gut bacteria, meaning their numbers increase
    - protect the mucous layer of the large intestine, to help prevent pathogens crossing the large intestine into the bloodstream
    - increase stool bulk, giving a mild laxative effect.

It is recommended that we consume around 30 grams of dietary fibre per day, or possibly more, from a combination of all three types. In Australia, most people have around 20 grams per day, but it is mostly roughage/insoluble fibre – many of us don't get anywhere near enough soluble fibre and resistant starch. Eating a variety of whole grains, fruit, vegetables and legumes makes it easy to get enough of the different fibre types.

WHAT IS PREBIOTIC DIETARY FIBRE?

Prebiotic fibre is a type of dietary fibre that passes, undigested, through to the large intestine, where the gut bacteria feeds on it (fermentation). Prebiotic fibre causes changes in the composition and activity of gut microbiota that have health benefits to the host (the person they live in). It is found in foods like underripe (green) bananas, onions, garlic, asparagus, oats (beta-glucan), legumes and BARLEYmax (a CSIRO-developed barley that can be found in commercial food products such as cereal and breads). Resistant starch is a type of prebiotic fibre. It is thought that we may need 20 grams of prebiotic fibre a day. Insoluble fibres are not fermented, but some soluble fibre has prebiotic activity.

The beneficial gases (short-chain fatty acids) produced by the fermentation of prebiotic fibre help increase the number of good bacteria, and keep bad bacteria numbers down.

I once introduced a high-prebiotic-containing breakfast cereal to one of the teams I was working with. I put a warning on the cereal dispenser: 'Take it slow.' Not being used to the load of dietary fibre, if players had a lot initially, the gas produced during fermentation would likely cause discomfort until their gut got used to it. It's important to increase dietary fibre intake gradually, especially the prebiotic and soluble types. A couple of staff members told me it got their bowels going, which was perfect. Probably not the best pre-game cereal, though ...

Sometimes people think they are healthy and active and therefore assume they don't need to worry about things like gut health, but as you can see, it is very important for overall health. We need all types of fibre to keep things moving along. Some to soften, some to bulk up and others to feed the bacteria that keep our gut happy.

TIPS FOR BOOSTING DIETARY FIBRE

To increase dietary fibre, I encourage the athletes I work with to choose wholegrain carbohydrates, e.g. wholegrain bread over white, and high-fibre breakfast cereals.

Remember, the variety of fibre types is just as important as the total amount. Try these tips to ensure you get the right amount and range of dietary fibre:

- Include fruit, preferably two servings per day, including the skin, e.g. kiwifruit, apples, pears, bananas.
- Have five servings of vegetables per day (which 93 per cent of Australians don't do, according to the latest Australian Health Survey 2011–12):
  - add more salad to your sandwich
  - add tomato, leafy greens and mushrooms to your breakfast eggs
  - cover one-third to half of your plate with vegetables at dinner
  - chomp on vegetables for snacks.
- Choose breakfast cereals with 7–8 grams or more of dietary fibre per 100 grams, and look out for those boasting a variety of dietary fibres, such as resistant starch.
- Use whole grains such as brown rice, freekeh and barley, and eat wholegrain bread.
- Have a handful of nuts per day (30 grams).
- Sprinkle a teaspoon or two of chia seeds on cereal or through yoghurt.

> - Add a sprinkle of seeds to your salad, cereal or stir-fry.
> - Include legumes or lentils in salads, soups or curries (they can cause bloating or excess gas at first, so add them gradually; things usually settle down after a few weeks, when your gut bacteria have started to settle back into shape).
> - Eat cooked, cooled potato, pasta, rice and stale bread (toasted).

At times, you may wish to modify your dietary fibre intake to include lower-fibre foods, such as choosing white bread over wholegrain, white rice over brown, eating a lower-fibre breakfast cereal or a ripe banana over a firm one. This would generally happen when carbohydrate energy is needed rapidly, such as when eating close to exercise, during an endurance event, and at half time during a match. It may also help when carbohydrate loading, as foods that are lower in dietary fibre are less filling, meaning you can eat more carbohydrate before you are full.

INCREASING FLUID FOR BOWEL HEALTH

Having enough fluid is essential for good stool form and frequency, particularly to avoid constipation. Around three-quarters of your stool is water, and the rest is made up of dietary fibre, bacteria and dietary fats. A high-fibre diet must include plenty of water for the fibre to soak up, otherwise it is a bit like making cement without enough water. Fluid is critical to a good poo.

Looking at your urine will help you determine if you have had enough to drink. It should be fairly clear in colour, like pale straw. (See page 64 for more about checking your hydration.)

TIPS FOR INCREASING YOUR FLUID INTAKE

- » Have a glass of water in the morning, either before or with breakfast.
- » After going to the toilet, grab a glass of water.
- » Drink water during and after exercise, and whenever you feel thirsty.
- » If you're not sure if you are hungry, try having a cup of tea, a glass of milk or a glass of water first – you may actually be thirsty.
- » Keep a jug of water on your desk, in the fridge or on the bench, and on the table at dinner.
- » Add mint leaves to your water, or sliced fruit (remembering it can be acidic, so watch for dental erosion).
- » Try drinking herbal teas.
- » Have a glass of milk for a snack.
- » Carry water when travelling, as this is a time when dehydration can be greater (especially on planes) and bowels can be less cooperative.

THE RISKS OF INTENSE EXERCISE TO IMMUNE FUNCTION

Ongoing intense exercise puts an athlete's immune system under stress. Emerging evidence suggests that changes in the gut can cause increased permeability. This can lead to a greater risk of infection.

During intense exercise, blood flow to the gut is reduced, while blood flow to the working muscles increases. This can damage the gut, allowing more pathogens to cross from the intestine into the bloodstream. Eating before and/or during exercise, particularly carbohydrate-containing foods, may counteract this by diverting some blood supply to the gut for digestion and absorption. Wearing compression garments can also increase blood supply to the gut, as they increase blood return (venous return) in the veins back to the heart, ready to be pumped out again.

Exercising in extreme heat, particularly if core body temperature rises, can also damage the lining of the gut. This can initiate an inflammatory response that gives the central nervous system (including the brain) the perception of fatigue. Acclimatising to training in the heat and adopting strategies for keeping the body cool are both essential to protect the gut. Cool beverages, slushies, ice vests and ice baths can all help. It is also important to cease exercise when it is too hot.

IMPROVING YOUR GUT MICROBIOTA

Your gut microbiota are the microorganisms or bacteria that live in the large intestine. They are influenced by what you eat, your lifestyle and your genetics. Your gut microbiota is as unique to you as your fingerprint. Dietary changes alter your gut microbiota, and a change in bacteria can occur within 24 hours of some dietary changes, with the aim of having a thriving, varied population of beneficial gut bacteria. We can measure these changes through faecal sample testing, which can identify and count the number of bacteria in your gut. This testing is becoming less expensive, so perhaps eventually looking at your gut bacteria will be as common as checking your cholesterol as a marker of health.

Good gut bacteria are very important for a healthy digestive system, and need looking after in order to thrive. See chapter 8, page 88, for more information about the benefits of good gut bacteria.

PROBIOTICS

You can add to your microbiota by consuming probiotics. Probiotics are live microorganisms (good bacteria) that live in the gut and have a health benefit when administered in adequate amounts. Probiotics are found in foods such as yoghurt, probiotic-containing drinks, fermented foods and oral probiotic supplements.

Probiotics can contain various strains. We are still learning about what these individual strains are best for – some may be more suited for improving regularity, others for immune health. Depending on what you are after, check claims for the various strains to make sure you are getting what you need. Research is still emerging, so it is best to try a product for a few weeks and see if it gives you the desired benefit. Another thought is that it may be best to work on improving the gut bacteria balance you have, rather than trying to introduce more or different strains. Further research needs to be done in this area.

Adding probiotic strains to your gut is not a one-off fix. If you want these bacteria to continue to live in your gut you need to add to them regularly, as often they may be different bacteria to your genetic make-up. Be sure to keep your prebiotic fibre intake up, too – the probiotics need feeding with prebiotics in order to prosper and grow.

TIPS FOR INCREASING GOOD GUT FLORA

- Eat a diet high in a range of dietary fibres – soluble, insoluble and resistant starch – to feed your gut bacteria, so they don't feed on you.
- Include probiotics from yoghurt or yoghurt-based drinks or probiotic milks. Check labels for probiotic strains and quantity (colony numbers). To be called a probiotic yoghurt, the product must contain at least 1 billion live microorganisms. Probiotic milks tend to have greater numbers and varieties of strains.
- You can try fermented foods from non-dairy sources such as sauerkraut and kimchi (Korean fermented vegetables). Look for unpasteurised, refrigerated varieties – commercially prepared sauerkraut is often made with vinegar and pasteurised, meaning that most bacteria will no longer be living. Food safety is important, so watch home brews of fermented products to ensure harmful bacteria are not present. Other foods such as miso and tempeh also contain beneficial bacteria.
- Watch the type of cooking oil you use, as some are better for the gut than others. The best options are those that promote anti-inflammatory effects, such as extra virgin olive oil.
- Limit saturated fat intake (e.g. processed snack foods, deep-fried foods, fat on meat). Don't overdo the meat.
- Cook extra pasta, rice and potatoes and freeze or refrigerate for the next meal. This will save time and increase the resistant starch levels.

- » To minimise gut inflammation and overall inflammation (important for athletes), increase your polyphenol antioxidant intake by eating fruit and vegetables, spices, tea, nuts, seeds and extra virgin olive oil. Sometimes active people can forget about the importance of these, as they concentrate on protein- and carbohydrate-containing foods. Benefits to gut health are a good motivator to pile some extra vegetables onto your plate.
- » Be careful not to eat too much protein – undigested proteins pass into the large intestine, where protein-fermenting bacteria eat them and produce noxious substances including ammonia. This can negatively affect the good bacteria populations, and will also produce smelly gas.
- » Grains in the diet are very important for oral gut bacteria (the mouth). Low-carbohydrate diets may reduce numbers of oral bacteria, which are responsible for nitrate to nitrite conversion. This opens blood vessels to allow more blood flow, which is important for blood pressure. Endurance athletes take supplements like beetroot juice due to the nitrate levels.
- » Eating a varied diet including plenty of plant foods is key to having a diverse gut bacterial colony.

I recommend that clients incorporate gut health–benefiting foods into their daily diets. This can be quite easy – have some yoghurt as part of a pre- or post-training snack (it also provides protein and calcium), throw in some nuts and fruit and your gut bacteria will be pretty happy.

There are a number of gut-related conditions, allergies and intolerances that can have an impact on our diet, wellbeing and sometimes performance. The following section will explore some of these.

FODMAP AND IRRITABLE BOWEL SYNDROME

When people suffer from bloating and general stomach or bowel discomfort, this is often diagnosed as irritable bowel syndrome (IBS). Until recently, not much was known to help with the symptoms. Now we understand much more, and dietary intervention can help relieve many of the symptoms.

As I have grown older, some of the foods I used to love, such as baked beans, now give me abdominal pain. This can be excruciating. For a while I cut out baked beans altogether, but then realised they offer a quick meal with important dietary fibre and protein. I have now learnt that how much and how often I eat these foods can make a difference. One slice of toast with baked beans is all I can handle – any more and I will pay for it. It is important to find your tolerance level, rather than cutting foods out altogether. Legumes like baked beans are a great source of soluble fibre and resistant starch that your bacteria can ferment. Restricting these foods severely could reduce the good bacteria levels in your gut.

When people restrict carbohydrate intake to follow a low-carbohydrate diet or to avoid the bloating that they attribute to certain carbohydrates, they can actually be negatively affecting their gut bacteria, making the whole issue worse!

There is a group of short-chain carbohydrates and sugar alcohols that are less able to be digested by some people. These pass into the large intestine, where they draw water into the gut and are fermented by bacteria-producing gas. This gas and extra fluid can cause gut distention, resulting in pain, bloating, abdominal discomfort, excess flatulence or wind, tiredness, and constipation, diarrhoea or both. Some people have nerves that are extra sensitive to the distention, and therefore experience pain. These short-chain carbohydrates and sugar alcohols are collectively referred to by the acronym FODMAP (fermentable oligosaccharides, disaccharides, monosaccharides and polyols). We can only touch on this briefly here, but Monash University is the leader in the FODMAP area, and has lots of great resources if you need further information.

If you are experiencing gut problems, these may be due to one or many FODMAP-containing foods. Modifying your diet to limit these foods can result in a significant improvement in symptoms. It's best not to cut out large amounts of foods long-term, however – the aim is to minimise symptoms while keeping your diet open to as many foods as possible. Seeking guidance from a health professional is best, particularly from an accredited practising dietitian. They will be able to help you work out which foods are causing your symptoms by cutting out high-FODMAP foods and then gradually reintroducing them to see what level of each food you can tolerate.

The types of foods that often need to be restricted are those with high:

- » **fructose**, e.g. pears, honey, mango, watermelon
- » **fructans**, e.g. artichokes, large quantities of garlic, wheat, rye and barley, inulin (a fibre often added to packaged foods), leek and onions
- » **lactose**, e.g. milk, some yoghurt, milk powder, soft cheese (ricotta, cottage, mascarpone)
- » **galacto-oligosaccharides (GOS)**, e.g. legumes and lentils
- » **polyols**, e.g. apples, apricots, plums, mushrooms, artificial sweeteners such as sorbitol (420), xylitol (967) and sugar alcohols such as maltitol (965) and mannitol (427).

Don't restrict these foods if you do not have any issues. Only people who experience undesirable symptoms may need to limit quantities.

FRUCTOSE MALABSORPTION

Have you heard someone say they are fructose intolerant? Fructose is one of the fermentable FODMAP carbohydrates that some people don't tolerate well, as it can cause bloating and excess flatulence. Fructose is naturally found in many fruits and honey, but can also be refined into syrups and added to processed sweet foods. If you are fructose intolerant, it is important to read the labels to check for fructose syrups.

A couple of years ago I worked with a football player who suffered from debilitating stomach cramps and bloating a few hours after breakfast, just before starting morning training. We changed his breakfast cereal, thinking it might have been the fructans in the wheat, and we cut out the fruit juice, which was high in fructose, but still the symptoms persisted. After further questioning I discovered he was adding honey to his cup of tea and to his cereal. He had swapped table sugar, which contains sucrose, for honey, thinking it would be a lower sugar option. But honey is pure sugar, too.

In this case, it was an inability to absorb the fructose in the honey that was causing his pain. He returned to having a small amount of sugar in his tea, and a low-fructose fruit such as banana or berries on his cereal, and his discomfort went away.

LACTOSE INTOLERANCE

Another of the fermentable carbohydrates that people can have an intolerance to is lactose. Lactose is the sugar that naturally occurs in milk. Lactose is made up of two sugar molecules: glucose and galactose. These must be split by the lactase enzyme in the small intestine in order to be digested. In people lacking the lactase enzyme, the lactose moves through to the large intestine where it draws in water, which can cause diarrhoea. Bacteria in the large intestine ferment the lactose, which can cause bloating from the gas produced. As we age, our ability to produce lactase can decrease, and lactose malabsorption can develop as a result.

Many people believe that you can't have dairy when you are lactose intolerant, but this is not the case. If you have an intolerance to the lactose in milk, use lactose-free milk, have small amounts only, or add a lactase enzyme to standard milk before drinking it (just follow the instructions on the lactase enzyme packaging).

Lactose-free cow's milk is milk that has had the lactase enzyme added, thus the lactose has been split and the individual sugar molecules can be absorbed. Though the sugar content is the same, lactose-free milk tastes sweeter. This is because the lactose has been split into glucose and galactose sugar molecules, giving more individual sugars to stimulate your tastebuds, as well as a combination of sugars that have sweeter taste profiles.

As milk and other dairy foods are a valuable, convenient source of nutrients for active people, I see them as a package deal of protein, carbohydrate, electrolytes and vitamins all in one. Don't cut them out if you don't need to.

ALMOND AND OTHER PLANT MILK ALTERNATIVES

There are many alternatives to cow's milk nowadays, and some people may not be aware of what they are buying. My first suggestion is not to compare them to each other. They have completely different nutrient profiles to dairy milk, which is not surprising, given that one is from an animal and the other a plant. Treat them as completely different foods, rather than alternatives.

If you are choosing not to have dairy milk and use an alternative plant-based beverage, it's important to think about where you will get your calcium from. Dairy is the main source of calcium for many people. Some beverages, such as soy and some almond milks, contain added calcium, which can be a good choice. Otherwise, you can get calcium from other areas of your diet, such as sesame seeds, broccoli, the bones of canned fish (sardines, salmon), and soy products.

To really know what you are buying, make sure you read the labels. Almond milk contains a varying percentage of almond, anything from 5 per cent to around 12 per cent. This means it might only have a handful of almonds in one litre, or five almonds per glass. That is expensive filtered water – it in no way replicates the nutritional value of eating almonds. Enjoy it as part of your diet if you like it, but be mindful of what the nutritional composition is.

For active people, it is important to compare the protein content of alternative milks. The protein content of almond milk (~0.5%), oat milk (~2.5%), quinoa milk (~0.5%) and rice milk (0.3%) are all low in comparison to cow's milk (4%). That is around 1.5 grams of protein in a 250 millilitre glass of almond milk, compared to 10 grams in cow's milk. Soy is higher in protein (3%), so is a better alternative if you need more protein in your diet. Read the labels and compare nutrition panels per 100 millilitres, as some products are starting to contain higher protein levels. Of course, other foods could be your major source of protein instead.

Many milk alternatives contain emulsifiers or gums that are not in cow's milk. These are not necessarily bad (however, some emulsifiers are being researched for possible adverse effects on gut bacteria) – they are needed to keep the nut or grain from separating out from the added water, and give a thicker, milk-like consistency. It is, however, important to realise that the milky thickness comes more from the added gums than from the product being packed full of almonds. Some almond milks contain sugar, so check this on the label too. If you are choosing almond milk for the nutritional benefits of almonds, eat a handful of almonds instead. If you are drinking it because you like it, because you want to mix your diet up, or because you're following a vegan diet, go for it – just be aware of the nutritional limitations.

Coconut milk has a great taste but is high in saturated fat – around 15 grams of fat per 100 millilitres, compared to full-cream cow's milk, which has 3.8 grams per 100 millilitres. You can buy lower fat coconut milks, which contain 7 grams per 100 millilitres. Consider frequency of use in the context of your whole diet.

Alternatives to cow's milk are great for increasing food options, particularly for people following vegan diets and those who have a digestive issue or an allergy to the protein in cow's milk. Just remember that they are nutritionally different.

A combination of milk and milk alternatives in your diet is great, too – you don't have to be loyal to one. Know what you are buying, what nutrients you are hoping for, and make informed choices.

IS GLUTEN FREE HEALTHIER FOR ME?

The answer is, it depends. Some people have a wheat intolerance. Eating gluten-free foods will relieve their symptoms because these foods are wheat free, and therefore do not contain the fermentable carbohydrate fructans – the benefit is not because they are gluten free. They could still be enjoying the health benefits and taste of other wheat-free foods that contain gluten, such as oats, rye and freekeh.

People with a wheat intolerance can usually eat foods containing wheat in small amounts, or a different wheat variety, such as spelt, because they have an intolerance, rather than an allergy. Be careful not to cut out food groups or narrow your food selection unnecessarily – this limits intake of valuable nutrients, particularly fibres for gut health.

It's important to examine a food for its total nutritional benefits. Gluten-free claims have become very popular with marketers, because many people incorrectly assume it must be a healthier alternative. A gluten-free diet is essential for people with coeliac disease, who have an abnormal immune response to gluten, the protein found in wheat, barley, oats and rye, which damages the small intestine. But for others removing gluten is of no benefit.

In fact, if we look at a wholefood, such as a gluten-free biscuit, made with rice flour, palm oil and sugar, we will see that it is high in saturated fat, high in sugar and low in dietary fibre. It's no healthier than a standard biscuit, and in some cases it's actually worse – a biscuit with oats (which contain gluten) may at least contain some fibre. The dietary fibre content of many gluten-free products is often lower than the gluten-containing equivalent. Breakfast cereals and breads are a good example of this, and are important foods for active people.

Gluten-free products are often more expensive. Why pay more for a product that could be nutritionally poorer?

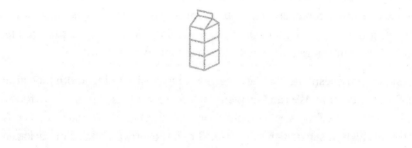

CHAPTER 10
Superfoods

How does a food achieve 'superfood' status? Is it if a celebrity has sworn by it? If it is rare and grown in an exotic location? There's no clear criteria for classifying a food as a 'superfood', but having a high antioxidant level and being very high in a particular nutrient are common characteristics.

Every vegetable is a superfood in my eyes, with the more variety the better. Plenty of other foods are super, too – nuts, seeds, seafood, eggs, legumes, whole grains, extra virgin olive oil, meats and dairy, too. All the food groups offer different things that benefit our health and performance.

A superfood doesn't need to be expensive or exclusive to the health food aisle or speciality store. We can buy plenty of common foods that are superfoods. They key to a healthy diet is usually more about the foods we leave out. Foods that are high in sugar, high in poor-quality fat, overly processed or packaged are not superfoods, and it's best to keep those portions small. Following is a breakdown of some of the most popular superfoods. Just remember, including one superfood in your diet is not going to make a big difference to your health or performance – you need plenty of them.

KALE

Kale is a fabulous green, leafy vegetable that is often classed as a superfood. However, I am somewhat turned off from using kale because it often costs twice as much as all the other green leafy vegetables, which are also superfoods in my eyes. (Admittedly, it is pretty hard to make spinach chips.)

I recommend a mixture of many super leafy greens – have fun with them. Try using spinach, silverbeet, cabbage, broccoli, and a variety of lettuce and beetroot leaves. Most contain vitamins A and C and folate, along with other antioxidants that are great for boosting the immune system. They're also all high in dietary fibre and low in kilojoules, due to their high water content.

Leafy greens are micronutrient (vitamin and mineral) powerhouses too, particularly iron, although not in an absorbable form until you eat a food that contains vitamin C (see page 90). They're a great choice for any vegetarian athletes and for anyone wanting to boost their iron intake. We can't exercise to our best with low iron stores – we need iron to carry the oxygen around our body.

Add any of the leafy greens to a smoothie, have them with eggs for breakfast, in your sandwich at lunchtime, in soup, stir-fries or as a side vegetable in the evening. Remember, people who exercise intensely put greater strain on their immune system, so it is important to eat plenty of vegetables to boost it.

BERRIES

Blueberries, goji and acai berries seem to have been granted superfood status, but raspberries, blackberries, strawberries, loganberries and cranberries are also packed with micronutrients, including anthocyanins, the antioxidant that gives berries and red grapes their dark red and purple pigment. Anthocyanins are known for their benefit to heart health, reducing oxidation of cholesterol that may otherwise form plaque on arterial walls.

Acai berries are labour-intensive to pick and need to be freeze-dried to prevent loss of nutrients from the flesh and skin. Most acai products therefore only contain a small amount of acai berry mixed with a lot of fillers such as maltodextrin, a carbohydrate made from processing starch. Maltodextrin is rapidly absorbed, like glucose. Be aware of what you are buying – your 'acai smoothie bowl' might actually be a maltodextrin bowl with just a splash of acai berry in the powder.

Cranberries are quite sour, so dried varieties are usually mixed with sugar. They are still healthy, however, and berries are a low-sugar fruit.

Frozen berries are snap frozen and often more economical, particularly if you are buying them out of season. I check to see where they were grown and aim for Australian where possible. Enjoy a variety of berries, fresh where possible, and buy them when they're in season so you don't break the bank.

SALMON

Salmon is a popular fish particularly high in omega 3 fats, known to be beneficial for heart and brain health. Along with an array of other nutrients such as B group vitamins, salmon is also high in the antioxidant astaxanthin, which gives salmon its deep red colour. Salmon, brown rice and broccoli is an incredibly popular combination, and for good reason. It's packed with good fats (omega 3) and protein from the salmon, high-fibre carbohydrates from the brown rice, antioxidants, vitamin C and more from the broccoli. And on top of all that, it tastes great.

If you don't like salmon, choose another type of fish or seafood. Sardines and mackerel, along with other oily fish, are also high in anti-inflammatory omega 3 fats. Levels vary depending on what the fish feed on, the type of fish, and the time of year.

I can remember my dad making sardines for breakfast with squeezed lemon and sliced tomato when we were young. We loved it! Sardines can take some getting used to, but nutritionally speaking, they're worth the effort (fresh sardines on the barbecue are quite delicious). I once prepared a range of sandwich items at Hawthorn and encouraged the players to try sardines, but there weren't many takers. With familiarisation I am sure they would have grown used to them.

ALMONDS

Almonds have become very popular over the years. I remember when they were the cheaper of the nuts. All types of nuts are packed with valuable vitamins, minerals, fibre, protein and fat, so enjoy a variety. Nuts have varying levels of different nutrients, so there's no need to stick to one kind. Try to have around a handful or so of nuts a day.

YOGHURT

Yoghurt is one of my favourite superfoods. I have it on my breakfast, with a salad, in a curry, in pumpkin soup, or for dessert. I just love it! The protein and calcium in the milk is super in itself, but what sets yoghurt apart is the probiotic cultures it contains. They help boost the growth of good bacteria in your gut and reduce the growth of pathogenic (bad) bacteria, giving you a stronger immune system. Some yoghurts contain minimal probiotic culture and lots of sugar, so look for yoghurts that are labelled 'probiotic yoghurt', and check the sugar levels based on your needs.

The bacteria in yoghurt breaks down lactose sugar, so people with a lactose intolerance can usually enjoy yoghurt. The protein in yoghurt helps keep you feeling full for longer, and is great for recovery after exercise.

Yoghurt is a great food to have before or after a training session. Aim to have around 20 grams of protein post-exercise. A 200-gram tub of yoghurt usually has around 10–12 grams of protein, although some new strained varieties on the market can contain up to 20 grams. Yoghurt also contains some carbohydrates (around 25–30 grams in a 200-gram serve, depending on the yoghurt), and minerals such as potassium and calcium, which have the added benefit of acting as electrolytes to aid rehydration.

LEGUMES

Although legumes may not be the most attractive-looking food, nutritionally speaking, they are very attractive. If I was giving out superfood ratings, legumes would rate very highly. They are cheap to buy, high in dietary fibre, protein and carbohydrate, and provide iron, zinc, magnesium and loads of other vitamins and minerals. Legumes are important in a vegetarian or vegan diet because of the nutrients they contain, including protein, iron and zinc. For athletes, legumes provide the perfect package deal for a recovery meal.

The high dietary fibre in legumes, together with the carbohydrate structure, means they have a low glycaemic index rating and are digested slowly, meaning your blood glucose level goes up gradually. They keep you full for longer and give you a slow release of energy, plus the soluble fibre they contain helps reduce cholesterol levels.

People sometimes avoid legumes because of the flatulence they can cause, but this is actually a good sign. Some of the dietary fibre and carbohydrate contained in lentils is fermented in the large intestine, producing gas. For some people this can cause discomfort, but that gas is good for your bowels and helps protect against bowel disease. To help reduce the discomfort of flatulence, try adding legumes gradually into your diet and watch what other ingredients you cook with them. If you have issues with FODMAP foods (see page 108), don't cook your legumes with onion and garlic, use small amounts, and avoid consuming them on consecutive days.

Rinsing canned legumes a few times helps remove some of the oligosaccharides – that's the 'sludge' you see in the can. This is made up of water, sometimes salt, and the carbohydrate that has come out of the beans. These oligosaccharides are sugars that end up in the large intestine, where they are fermented, producing gas. If you don't mind that 'sludge' in canned legumes, save it and put it in soups for flavour. You can even whip up the sludge from canned chickpeas instead of egg whites to make a pavlova, or anything that would usually call for whipped egg whites. You can freeze canned legumes if you don't use them all in one go.

If your family complain about the flatulence, just tell them it's part of your 'gut health' program.

There's plenty more I could say about superfoods, but you get the picture – plant foods and minimally processed foods feature highly, so load up on these. Like fashion, superfoods cycle in and out of popularity. Our tastes can work in the same way, loving a food for a while before overdosing on it and then moving on to the next food. The most important thing is that you are meeting your nutritional needs and enjoying your food.

SECTION 2

EATING FOR PERFORMANCE AND RECOVERY

CHAPTER 11

What Should I Eat Before Exercise?

What to eat before exercise varies enormously depending on what kind of exercise you are doing and for how long, what time of the day it is, and what your goals and individual preferences are.

THE GLYCAEMIC INDEX

Eating lower glycaemic index (GI) foods can be beneficial when looking for a sustained energy release. This could be lower-intensity exercise lasting for more than 60 minutes, such as a long bike ride, surfing for several hours, playing golf, cross-country skiing and hiking. Individuals playing sports that require concentration and precision, such as archery and shooting, may also benefit from eating lower-GI carbohydrates, because they take time to be digested and provide a gradual supply of energy.

Low-GI foods such as legumes, porridge (cooked oats) and dense wholegrain breads may be too heavy in the stomach to eat just before intense training. Have these 2 hours or so prior to exercise. Runners often prefer higher GI foods to avoid gut upset.

Most people will benefit from eating some carbohydrate 1–4 hours before exercising. A small percentage of people who eat high-GI carbohydrates in the hour before exercise experience a metabolic response that causes a dip in blood glucose levels, resulting in rapid onset of fatigue at the beginning of exercise and symptoms similar to hypoglycaemia (low blood sugar level, feeling light-headed and shaky). It is very individual – trial and error will help you determine what is best for you.

DO I NEED TO EAT BEFORE MORNING EXERCISE?

Whether you need to eat before morning exercise depends on a number of factors.

When making this decision, ask yourself:

- » How hungry am I when I wake up? Will I feel fatigued during exercise if I don't eat beforehand?
- » Will I feel too heavy if I eat before morning exercise, given that there won't be sufficient time for the food to start to digest?
- » What did I eat the night before? Did it contain a significant amount of carbohydrate to fuel this session?
- » How did I feel last session? Did I have enough energy? (Remember, many factors will influence this.) What did I eat? Did this fuel me adequately without leaving me feeling too heavy?

Listening to your body and experimenting will help you find what works best for you.

Most people don't need to eat before a 30-minute morning walk. If you have low blood glucose levels and/or diabetes, the case may be different, but the rest of us should have plenty of stored fuel reserves. In most cases, a drink prior to the session and breakfast when you return will suffice. That doesn't mean you can't eat beforehand if you would prefer to, though.

Someone undertaking early morning swimming training that covers 3+ kilometres, including sprints, would benefit from some fuel such as toast or a banana and a glass of milk, because this provides protein, carbohydrate, fluid and electrolytes. A small snack during training (sultanas, mouthfuls of fruit or muesli bar, a sports drink) is an alternative method of keeping energy levels up if little can be eaten prior.

No-one wants to wake up an hour earlier to leave time for digestion when you are already getting up early for training. If you have replenished fuel stores after the previous day's training session, you should have adequate fuel stores for the morning training (and you can top up during training if you are doing a long session). Pre-training breakfast is more about topping up blood glucose levels, providing some protein and satisfying hunger. A fruit smoothie, a tub of yoghurt, a piece of toast or a mug of soup are good options for those who struggle to eat much before early morning training.

ENERGY REQUIREMENTS: WEIGHT GAIN, MAINTENANCE OR REDUCTION?

Your daily energy requirements should be considered when deciding how much you need to eat before exercise. If you are exercising to help with weight management or loss, then perhaps include what you eat prior to exercise as part of your daily intake, rather than adding extra. You can move food around in the day to fuel your session. Timing is everything!

You might:

» split breakfast in half and have some before and some after a morning session

» have two lunches – one around 11.30 am and the other around 3 pm – rather than lunch and a morning and afternoon snack

» have your afternoon snack (or second lunch) around 2 hours before afternoon training. A lower GI lunch that also includes protein would be perfect for this, such as a quinoa and boiled egg salad, tuna and noodles with vegetables, a salad and lean beef sandwich, or mixed beans with corn and greens. Doing this means you are fuelling yourself for the session without adding in extra food.

If, on the other hand, you need to maintain weight or gain muscle mass, then your pre-training eating needs to provide extra food intake to help prevent a deficit resulting from energy burnt during exercise. Early morning exercise might include breakfast both before and after. I work with many rowers who grab a bowl of cereal before getting on the water and have eggs with avocado on toast afterwards. Think about some carbohydrate for energy and protein that can contribute to muscle mass growth and repair. If you have some protein in your system, your body is more likely to reduce the catabolic (breakdown) state and increase the anabolic (building) state, which is important for muscle gain.

'TRAINING LOW'

In recent years some athletes have been experimenting with 'training low'. This means training in a fasted or low-carbohydrate state for some of their training sessions. They might do this to help manage body composition by getting their body to burn more fat and spare carbohydrate. Their overall diet isn't low in carbohydrate, just the meals before exercise.

To train low (sometimes referred to as 'sleeping low') you complete a heavy training session so you are carbohydrate depleted, have an evening meal that's low in carbohydrate, and then exercise in the morning either without eating, or after eating a breakfast that does not contain carbohydrate.

Research doesn't show the performance benefits from 'training low' that many people might expect. Metabolic changes may occur, with the body burning more fat than carbohydrate. In ultra-endurance events, where fat can be an adequate fuel supply, this adaptation could theoretically result in greater energy availability, by sparing carbohydrate. The performance issue occurs when the intensity increases, such as when sprinting up a hill or to the finish line. High-intensity exercise requires carbohydrate. If carbohydrate stores are still low and haven't been replenished, there will be insufficient fuel to accelerate to the finish line. This is an important consideration if following a long-term low-carbohydrate intake.

If you are considering 'training low', understand that during training you are likely to experience lower energy levels, a greater perception of effort and an increase in stress to the immune system. It is not advisable to 'train low' for an intense training session too often or without consideration and reason. Decide what the goal of these training sessions is and pick which, if any, are appropriate to train low. Speak with an accredited sports dietitian to determine when and if 'training low' will be of any benefit.

WHAT TO AVOID EATING BEFORE EXERCISE

- » Avoid eating very high-fat foods before exercise, as they are slow to digest and can make you feel lethargic. You want blood flow heading mostly to your muscles for exercise, rather than to your stomach to digest the fats. A small amount, such as a handful of nuts, a quarter or half an avocado, a slice of cheese or two would all be appropriate. A bucket of deep-fried chips, fried chicken, creamy sauces or a pastry item, on the other hand, would not be my recommended choices.
- » It can also be best to limit very high-fibre foods within the hour before exercise, as they take time to digest and could have you feeling overfull. This is most relevant if your exercise involves running or jumping around.
- » Overeating of anything can leave you feeling sluggish.
- » Drinking excess fluid just before exercise leaves it sitting in your stomach. Drink throughout the day instead.

LOOK AFTER YOUR GUT DURING EXERCISE

Having something to eat before long, intense exercise sessions will continue blood flow to your gut during the session (see chapter 9 for more on gut health). This may be protective to the gut wall, reducing its permeability and keeping pathogens (bad bacteria) from crossing through into the bloodstream. If you feel you can't eat before exercise, practise, and train your gut to handle having something in it, even if it is just a small amount of food and fluid, when exercising. Keep practising and experimenting during training. Rather than overeating so you feel discomfort, just have a small amount of food – you can top up during or after if needed.

ARE LOLLIES SUITABLE?

Lollies provide lots of carbohydrate in the form of sugar, but very few other nutrients. Wholefoods that provide nutrients as well as carbohydrate, such as B group vitamins B1, B2 and B3, which are involved in converting carbohydrate into energy, make better choices before and after exercise. During exercise lasting longer than 90 minutes, lollies can be an easy-to-eat carbohydrate food, but at other times we can easily choose foods that are much more nourishing to our overall health, such as:

- wholegrain bread with cheese or peanut butter/100 per cent nut spread
- cereal or muesli with yoghurt or milk
- fresh seasonal fruit (in-season food always tastes best)
- smoothie (fruit, milk or veggie base)
- soup
- rice paper rolls
- dried fruit and nut mixes.

In general, I recommend eating something within a few hours before exercising. That might mean moving a meal to fit into this time or adding in an extra one, depending on your energy needs. The idea of eating before exercise is to meet your individual needs and to fuel you so you get the most out of your exercise. What and how much you need will depend on your goal for the training session.

Now that we have before exercise sorted, what do we do during exercise?

CHAPTER 12

What to Eat on Game Day

You've put in the hard training and now it's showtime! Everything you do is with the aim of achieving optimum performance. Planning your intake for competition or game day means thinking about the food you'll eat and the fluid you'll drink before, during and after the event. Chapter 11, 'What Should I Eat Before Exercise?' (page 123), and chapter 13, 'Strategies for a Speedy Recovery' (page 139) also cover principles that can be applied to eating for competition.

When preparing for game day, we need to ensure we fuel and hydrate optimally. Running out of fuel or becoming dehydrated will diminish your ability to achieve your best.

With events lasting less than 30 minutes the aim is to start well fed and watered, and then not interfere with the task. Anything taken in during the event is not for performance benefit but for comfort, such as water to overcome a dry mouth or thirst.

HOW DOES COMPETITION EATING DIFFER TO OTHER TIMES?

The food we eat during competition has a short-term purpose, and may not be as nutritious as foods chosen at other times. Factors such as the food feeling light, being easy to digest and 'sitting well' in the stomach, along with what is available and practical, all significantly influence our food choices during competition. At other times, our nutritional needs, which influence health and wellbeing long-term, are most important.

On game day in AFL, I offer the players foods such as pikelets with jam. These foods are low in overall nutritional value, and they're not something I would recommend at other times, but they are easily digestible carbohydrates (high GI, low fibre), easy to eat and prepare in the change rooms, and don't require refrigeration. They can be eaten before, during or after a game, and the players like the taste. At other times I would encourage athletes to choose something more nutritious and lower in refined carbohydrate. Competition day foods are often not the things you should eat at other times.

GETTING READY FOR GAME DAY: CARBOHYDRATE LOADING

Carbohydrate loading is a technique used by athletes who are competing in events lasting longer than 90 minutes. The duration of carbohydrate loading will depend on the athlete, the intensity and the duration of the event. Endurance athletes who already eat a moderate- to high-carbohydrate diet may only need to increase levels the day before and on competition day. People less well trained may need to increase carbohydrate intake a few days prior.

Carbohydrate intake can vary between 7 and 13 grams of total carbohydrate per kilogram of body weight per day. It's best to consult an accredited sports dietitian to help you work out what your needs are. Experience, as well as what has worked for you in the past, is also important to consider.

Increasing carbohydrate intake results in extra water being stored by the body. Carbohydrate stores water with it as glycogen, therefore increased carbohydrate intake can often result in an increase in body weight. This is particularly important to consider in sports that have weight category restrictions. Carbohydrate loading can make some people feel heavier and bloated. AFL players, for example, prefer to feel light and fast on game day. It is important to strive for a happy medium between fuelling and feeling good.

If carbohydrate loading is important to ensure adequate fuel is stored for the event, lower-fibre carbohydrate foods can be handy. These are less filling, so you can eat a greater volume to meet your carbohydrate requirements. Salad and low-carbohydrate vegetables can take a back seat for these last meals to make room for the higher-carbohydrate foods. This may also reduce the need for a bowel motion at critical times.

People with conditions such as diabetes should seek specific advice before changing their carbohydrate intake.

GAME-DAY FOOD CONSIDERATIONS

Ask yourself the following questions when planning your game-day food arrangements:

- » **Food availability:** Will food be provided for you? Even if it will be, consider taking your own. Tennis player CoCo Vandeweghe refused to go back on court during the 2018 Australian Open because her banana wasn't ready for her between sets. She said she needed her potassium. If certain foods are important to you for psychological and/or physiological benefit, then don't take the risk of them not being available. In big events, it's best to be prepared.
- » **Be prepared:** What kind of food will be available to buy at the venue? I recommend taking your own – it's always best to have a backup option with you. The last thing you want to do is get stuck waiting in line, have trouble finding out where to buy food from or, even worse, find that they have run out.
- » **Facilities:** What preparation facilities will you have available? Does the food need to be prepared at home and taken with you (e.g. sandwiches to eat during a swim meet that goes all day)? Is refrigeration available? If not, it's important to pack food in a cooler bag with ice, and to consider the choice of fillings in sandwiches. Meats and dairy products need to be kept cold if they will be out of the fridge for more than a few hours. Cool drinks are more palatable to most people when exercising – freezing some bottles can work well.
- » **Practicalities:** Think about the practicality of the foods and fluids you're bringing. If you'll be riding, for example, how will you carry the

food and eat it? (You could cut sandwiches up in quarters and place them in the back pockets of your top.) If long-distance swimming, will there be a support crew to carry your food, prepare it and give it to you? If so, you may need to brief them. How do you swim and eat or drink? Always practise in training to determine how a food will work for you. Running and drinking at the same time is a skill. I tried this during a triathlon once, and more water ended up my nose than in my mouth!

» **Opportunity to eat:** What opportunity is there during the event to eat or drink? You will need to be extra diligent about hydration in a sport that offers minimal opportunity to drink while competing.

Some people prefer to eat minimally before competition. If it is a short, explosive event lasting less than a few minutes, such as a sprint, discus or javelin, adequate preparation can ensure you have enough energy without having to eat prior. If you have eaten well the day before to ensure adequate carbohydrate and fluid levels, and have eaten something 4 hours prior, this should be sufficient. It is recommended that you do keep up fluids, however.

Other athletes get hungry and don't like that feeling, so they choose to eat a small meal or snack to top up before the event. Work out what foods suit you and stick to that.

» **Gastrointestinal issues:** Is gastrointestinal discomfort an issue for you? Think about how certain foods make you feel, e.g. heavy, bloated and lethargic, or light, fast and fuelled. A big bowl of porridge an hour or less before an event could be too heavy – it won't have been fully digested before you compete. A smaller bowl of porridge or a moderate-sized bowl of a lower-fibre and higher-GI cereal such as wheat biscuits or flakes will be digested more quickly.

» **Liquid meals:** Liquid meals before competition work well for some people, as they are digested more quickly than solids. Others find the feeling of liquid moving around in their stomach unpleasant. Timing is important here. If you have the liquid meal (e.g. a smoothie) early enough before the event, it should be digested in time.

PRE-EVENT MEAL

Determining the right pre-event eating follows similar principles to deciding what to eat before exercise. Some extra considerations include:

» Are you competing in a contact sport? If so, having too much in your stomach might not agree with you.

» Is the event short, such as a swimming or running sprint event, where your warm-up will be longer than the event itself? In that case, you may prefer to feel light. Have your last main meal 3–4 hours prior to the event and top up with high-GI foods that will fuel you, but not leave you feeling heavy. You might have some porridge for breakfast 4 hours prior to competing, then closer to the event have a ripe banana, a wholemeal (rather than wholegrain) bread sandwich or handful of pretzels.

» What time does the event commence? If it's early in the morning, you don't want to sacrifice sleep and get up 4 hours earlier to eat. Instead, top up with a snack the night before, have a lighter breakfast, and then top up during or close to the event. Lower fibre, lower fat and moderate to lower protein foods will be more quickly digested, and are advisable if you are eating close to the event and are prone to gastrointestinal disturbances. A smoothie, a tub of yoghurt or a slice of toast with Vegemite could be good options here.

In the AFL the timing of matches changes, from day to afternoon to night. The same principles of timing work no matter what time the game is: eat the last meal around 3 hours beforehand, and then top up in the 2 hours before the game, with minimal food in the last hour. Keep up fluids throughout. As Aussie Rules is a contact sport, having too much food in your stomach can be uncomfortable. For example, a 2 pm game would involve breakfast around 8 am, a salad and meat roll around 11 am–12 pm, a muesli bar and a banana or other fruit around 1 pm, and fluid throughout.

Endurance events may require carbohydrate loading days prior, with the pre-event meal being consumed to top up muscle glycogen levels and hydration and to prevent hunger.

Eating carbohydrate food before exercise won't cause a sudden spike and then drop in blood glucose levels for most people. Eating and drinking carbohydrate might increase insulin levels, resulting in a metabolic change to burn more carbohydrate, but this has not been shown to affect performance. Any insulin increase would be small, and can be overcome by ensuring that enough carbohydrate has been eaten or drunk to compensate.

WHAT TO EAT DURING COMPETITION

For events lasting less than 60 minutes, you won't generally need to eat during the event. If you have multiple short events in one day, however, you may need to eat in between them. Continue to drink to offset fluid losses at a comfortable rate for all events.

Many team sports have quarter or half-time breaks, during which food and fluid can be taken in. Practise what you eat during breaks, as you will not have sufficient time for the food or fluid to be digested before you return to play. You can train your stomach to feel comfortable with some food and fluid in it. Low-fat and moderate-to-low-protein and -fibre foods will be digested more quickly. Fruit is often a good choice here. It provides carbohydrate, water and potassium, an electrolyte that aids with hydration.

Working out how much carbohydrate you need and what type, e.g. glucose, fructose or a mix, can be confusing. Glucose, glucose polymers and sucrose are all absorbed quite rapidly to maintain blood glucose levels. Fructose, on the other hand, is absorbed relatively slowly, and via a different transport mechanism. Including both glucose and fructose in a product means there are two different pathways of absorption, and therefore more carbohydrate for the body. When glucose and fructose are consumed together the glucose accelerates the absorption of fructose. Fructose is stored in the liver, mostly as liver glycogen.

Multiple types of carbohydrate, such as a mix of glucose, fructose and longer-chain carbohydrates (e.g. maltodextrins), can be an advantage for fluid reabsorption. Using longer-chain glucose polymers, rather than many individual glucose molecules, means the osmolality (concentration of molecules) of the solution will not increase. This is advantageous because it means the absorption of fluid will be more rapid into the bloodstream.

If the osmolality increases too much (when there are too many individual molecules in the fluid), water will move into the small intestine, to try and reduce the osmolality, rather than being absorbed into the bloodstream, causing gastrointestinal bloating and discomfort and slowing rehydration.

Sports gels and some sports drinks often contain a mix of different types of carbohydrates to increase the total carbohydrate that can be absorbed, and to maximise the hydration rate, keeping osmolality at the optimal level. Fruit sugars are a mix of carbohydrate types, glucose and fructose, making them a suitable snack for exercise.

In events lasting 2 hours or more the body needs a supply of carbohydrate to fuel performance. How much you need varies greatly depending on exercise intensity. It is estimated that around 30–60 grams of carbohydrate per hour is required for long events, and up to 90 grams per hour for those longer than 2.5 hours. Knowing the carbohydrate content of foods and fluids allows you to calculate the quantities needed and to space them out over the event.

Competitors in short events lasting 30–45 minutes may benefit from carbohydrate swirling. This involves swirling a drink containing carbohydrate in the mouth for around 5 seconds. The carbohydrate is noted by receptors in the mouth, which then signal to the brain that carbohydrate is available. You can then spit the fluid out. This can be done at regular intervals. The body's recognition of the carbohydrate seems to result in high physical output being sustained for longer, even though the carbohydrate was not swallowed. This may be useful for those who don't want to eat or ingest fluid, but need to boost energy levels. It is best suited to short events.

GAME-DAY PRACTICALITIES

When will you eat and drink during competition, and how will you do it? Does the sport allow you to drink freely? For example, during a marathon, drink aid stations are set up along the course. In football (soccer) there is limited opportunity to drink during play, whereas in AFL players can drink at just about any time, with trainers coming out constantly to bring them drinks.

When running long distances, food and fluid needs to be suitable to consume while on the move. It may have to be left outside at fuelling stations unrefrigerated. Fuel can be a particular challenge during long-distance swimming – it can be hard to swim and chew at the same time. I had a client whose spouse was part of the support crew for his ocean swims, and she would pre-chew jelly beans before handing them over to him.

Practise before race day. You need to know that your food choices will work for you. After consuming numerous gels during a long event, you may suffer from flavour fatigue, so make sure you pack a variety, including some salty and some sweet. Moist foods are easier to eat, particularly if your mouth is dry. Think about packaging, too – is it easy to open and get the food out? Take equipment to keep your food and fluid cool. If travelling to unknown places, take your own supply. It is important to have familiar foods available that you know work for you.

GAME-DAY HYDRATION

Deciding how much and what to drink at any time is very individual, and the type of activity plays a big role.

- » How long is the event?
- » Will fluid be available during the event, and if so, what kind?
- » Can I drink while competing?

The weather on the day of competition will also influence quantity and choice. Hawthorn once played on a cold day down in Tasmania, and one player was so cold post-game that I had to find him a hot chocolate drink to warm him up. On other days it can be scorching, and players need ice and cold drinks. Remember, even when it is cold, you still need to drink.

Given that you are unlikely to drink enough during competition to meet sweat losses, it is important to start the day well hydrated. Look at your urine colour – it should be the colour of pale straw. If you are regularly going to the toilet and your urine is the colour of water, you can probably back off a bit. You may need to consider adding some electrolyte-containing drinks to your fluid intake, not just plain water. Be careful not to drink to the point where you feel bloated.

To help achieve optimal hydration for competition day, ensure your rehydration practices replace fluid losses adequately. Experiment during training sessions. If you have had to dehydrate somewhat to 'make weight' for a sport, then rehydration before competition is important. Make sure you have a plan in place so you know how much fluid you need to lose and how you will replace this. Downing litres of water straight after weigh-in will result in frequent toilet trips, as much of the water will simply be lost as urine. The urge to go to the toilet can be disruptive to performance.

Excess fluid may be a disadvantage in sports where power to weight ratio is important. Excess weight can impede speed, change of direction or acceleration. In Formula One car racing, the amount of fluid the driver can carry is dependent on their weight and that of the car. Mark Webber, being a tall man for the sport, was relatively heavy, and was therefore restricted in the amount of fluid he could carry in the car. Imagine enduring the extreme heat in the car, wearing a fireproof suit and feeling thirsty while having to maintain extreme concentration. This limitation meant Mark's fluid requirements needed to be calculated and planned out carefully and accurately.

Your hydration needs to suit your sweat rate and concentration (we all have different amounts of salt and other electrolytes in our sweat). If your sweat is high in salt, you may need to drink numerous bottles of fluid on competition day, some with water and others with electrolyte-containing drinks to replace salt (electrolyte) losses. If your energy requirements are high on the day, the drink may need to provide carbohydrate as well. This is where sports drinks are suitable. While competing, and when you are fatigued, it is easier to drink than to eat.

Planning your fluid requirements and knowing what your needs are for competition is important. This will change with intensity and climate. If you don't have a hydration plan, it's easy to get caught up in the event and find that you have forgotten to drink and are already dehydrated to the point of impairing performance. For example, if you will be cycling a long distance, plan how many bottles of fluid you will need over a certain number of kilometres or time frame. You don't want to play catch-up and have large volumes of fluid sitting in your stomach.

Drinking electrolyte-containing drinks helps retain fluid and drive thirst. See chapter 5 (page 63) for more tips about hydration.

PRIMING THE STOMACH WITH FLUID

Having some fluid in the stomach before and during competition can aid with rehydration. The fluid causes distention of the abdomen, which increases the rate of gastric emptying to the small intestine, where the fluid is absorbed. Around 300 millilitres is a comfortable amount for most people to drink before exercise.

THE TRAP OF OVEREATING AND -DRINKING ON GAME DAY

Most sports are not long enough for you to run out of fuel. For example, an Aussie Rules game lasts for around 2 hours, and a netball game is 60 minutes, and players are able to eat and drink during the game. The meals leading up to the game, such as dinner the night before, breakfast in the morning and the meal or snack a few hours prior don't need to be so large that you will feel full and heavy. You don't need to carbohydrate load to the point of feeling overfull. There are plenty of opportunities to continually top up.

The right food and fluid intake on competition day will benefit performance. You need to determine what best suits your needs. Practise the timing and content of your food and fluid intake, and avoid trying new strategies on game day, but remain flexible, too. Environmental conditions, the food and drink available, and how you feel can all change. It is good to have routine that can also be flexible.

CHAPTER 13

Strategies for a Speedy Recovery

Recovery nutrition aims to restore losses caused by exercise and to prepare the body for the next session. It is not an excuse to eat everything in sight without thought. For optimal recovery, there are nutritional needs to consider beyond the kilojoules burnt during exercise. Find your balance.

Whether an elite athlete or a recreational one, your recovery needs are individual to you. There is no one-size-fits-all approach, and your own approach will also vary between sessions, such as adjusting how much protein and carbohydrate you have in your recovery meal. Asking yourself what the goal of each recovery meal is while also considering your overall nutrition needs is a good place to start.

DETERMINING YOUR RECOVERY NEEDS

Here are questions to ask yourself when determining your recovery needs:

- » What have I lost and how much (fluid, electrolytes, fuel)? In answering this question, consider the duration and intensity of the training session:
    - » Was this a big one?
    - » Weather conditions – did I sweat a lot?
- » How quickly do I need to restore the losses?
    - » What is the recovery time available between sessions?

- » Do I want to restore everything – all the energy and fluid used?
  - » If you are wanting to reduce body weight to meet a body weight category, for example, do you want to replace all energy used, or make an energy deficit in order to reduce weight?
  - » Will you need to be slightly dehydrated to make the weight category upon weigh-in in later in the day?
  - » Do you need to reduce body fat or muscle mass?
  - » If you are going to compete in a very hot environment, you may wish to train in a somewhat dehydrated state on occasion, to help you acclimatise to hot weather.
- » Do I want to take in extra energy so I have some 'spare'? You might need this for a variety of reasons, including:
  - » for muscle gain
  - » to load up for a future long session
  - » after the last training session before a match/competition/race.

Here are some examples:

- » There is little need for speedy recovery after a 4-hour marathon if you are taking the following two weeks off as rest, because there is a long time between sessions.
- » If you've just completed an intense 3-hour bike ride and you have training again the next day, recovery is very important and time-critical to ensure you get all the fuel in before the next session.
- » If you play a 90-minute football (soccer) game once a week, and also have training sessions that need to be recovered from during the week, then recovery is important, but you have the luxury of a little time. Perhaps you might complete a light training session the day before a game, then take in more than the food and fluid losses from the session in order to load for the game.
- » A person training for a triathlon who swims in the morning and wants to run or ride in the afternoon needs to recover from the swim to ensure they have optimal energy stores for the afternoon. They would look to refuel (carbohydrate), rehydrate (fluid, electrolytes) and repair/rebuild (protein, vitamins and minerals) quickly.

- » If competing in numerous short events over the day at a competition such as a swimming carnival, you will require tailored recovery between each event. Recovery after one swim is not critical, but when accumulating swims over the day it is. Also consider the training completed during the week prior. Recovery is essential.
- » If you complete two hour-long classes at the gym each week with days in between to recover, the next meal should be sufficient for recovery for most people. If needing to achieve weight gain, recovery food to supply extra energy is critical.

OVERDOING IT WITH RECOVERY FOOD AND FLUID

Some exercise sessions, such as a 45-minute class at the gym, don't require any 'special' recovery other than water, as energy and fluid losses are not significant. I listen to the frustrations of people trying to reduce body weight, complaining about how hard they have been exercising without achieving the desired results. When I ask about their food intake they tell me about shakes they have made to have before and after training, and the snacks they have also eaten for recovery. I give them the good and bad news. The good news is that by cutting out some of those unnecessary drinks and extra snacks, they should see results. The bad news is that they've been spending a lot of money on extras that have probably sabotaged their goals.

These people are often taking in more kilojoules than they need, sometimes more than they are burning during exercise. The body is efficient, and doesn't burn as many kilojoules as people often think. To gain muscle mass and possibly extra total mass, add in extra food and fluid for kilojoules. But those who are exercising at moderate or low intensity, or even high intensity but for short periods of time, and only a few hours a week, should use their daily food intake for recovery. There is no need for extra. Just adjust the timing of the food you would usually have to fuel and recover from the workout. This is further discussed in chapter 11, 'What Should I Eat Before Exercise?' (see page 123).

CARBOHYDRATE AND RECOVERY

The body is very efficient at replacing carbohydrate stores, particularly in the first hour to hour and a half post-exercise, and this then continues for another 12–24 hours. If your next training session is not far away then consuming carbohydrate within the first hour after exercise will start the process of recovery quickly, and will maximise your energy stores for the next session. This is particularly relevant for people training in the morning and then again in the afternoon. Early carbohydrate intake post-exercise is less critical if you have more than 12 hours to recover. However, delaying carbohydrate for more than 2 hours post-exercise after glycogen depletion is not recommended. Glycogen is the fuel stored as glucose in the muscle, and glycogen restoration will be very slow until feeding starts.

If your goal is to increase muscle mass, then starting your recovery early with carbohydrate and protein is beneficial. If you are not trying to gain weight and your next session is low intensity and/or a few days away, however, there is no rush. Your next meal containing some carbohydrate can replace the energy, topping up muscle and liver glycogen stores.

For the serious athlete, it is recommended that around 1 gram of carbohydrate per kilogram of body weight is eaten in the first meal or snack after exercise, generally within the first hour. I recommend that the footballers I work with eat between 50 and 100 grams (depending on body weight) of carbohydrate in the first hour after exercise. They then follow up with a meal containing carbohydrate in the following few hours.

In that first hour, a substantial part of the carbohydrate intake comes from fluids such as sports drinks, milk or smoothies, as they are easy to drink and help restore fluid balance. Sports drinks are generally drunk after intense exercise; at other times they are not generally required. For general training, food can be eaten afterwards to provide carbohydrate and electrolytes, along with valuable nutrients to contribute to an overall healthy diet. In those cases, water should be the main fluid.

Sometimes the need for fast-acting, high-GI carbohydrate for recovery can be seen as a justification for making high-sugar, low-nutrient choices, such as lollies, soft drink, sports drinks and biscuits. The negative effects of sweet drinks and lollies on teeth, for example, should be considered, as this is an issue for everyone, regardless of their fitness level or body weight. Overall health needs to be considered, particularly for athletes with frequent, sometimes twice-daily, sessions. Remember to choose food that will give you the best nutritional bang for your buck.

PROTEIN AND RECOVERY

Eating protein before and after exercise can help ensure that your body is in the building (anabolic) rather than breakdown (catabolic) phase. The circulating amino acids in the bloodstream pre-exercise help promote muscle growth. Having a meal with protein after exercise will aid with maintenance and building of muscle, reducing muscle soreness and inflammation while also benefiting the immune system.

Food eaten close to finishing exercise (generally within 1–2 hours) should contain around 20–30 grams of protein. This should be followed up again in the next 2–3 hours with usual meals and snacks thereafter.

Dr Stuart Phillips, whose research focuses on the impact of nutrition and exercise on human skeletal muscle protein turnover, recommends consuming 0.3–0.4 grams of protein per kilogram of body weight, 4–5 times per day, particularly for those aged 40 years and over, and 0.4 grams or more for those athletes aged 80+ years (see also page 50). More research is being conducted to determine the ideal protein intake for maintaining muscle mass as we age. We will look at this in more detail in chapter 14 (see page 151).

If exercising recreationally without wanting to increase muscle mass and with 24+ hours between sessions, there is no need to add in extra meals or snacks for recovery. Waiting until your next meal is sufficient. It is important to ensure adequate protein in this meal or snack to help meet your overall protein requirements for the day.

Always ensure you are having sufficient protein, particularly in snacks, where it can be lacking. Adding a glass of milk, a tub of yoghurt, extra seeds, nuts, canned fish or legumes or hard-boiled eggs are great easy ways to boost the protein in your diet.

FLUIDS AND RECOVERY – REHYDRATION

Work on replacing fluid lost during exercise. Weigh yourself (in underwear only) before and after the session and calculate the difference in weight. Add an extra 25–50 per cent to this figure due to sweating, which continues post-exercise, and for fluid already lost to urine in the bladder. This will give you a reasonable guide to how much fluid you have lost, and therefore how much you will need to drink for rehydration. For example, if you lose 2 kilograms, then you will need to drink 2.5–3 litres of fluid (see also page 66).

How quickly you need to rehydrate will depend on when your next training session is. If it is in a few days there is no great rush, but if it is within 12 hours, rehydrating more rapidly is important.

To be well hydrated at the end of the day, aim to drink enough fluid to ensure that you have fairly clear urine just before you go to bed, but not so much that you get up to go the toilet regularly, disrupting your sleep. Sometimes high sweat losses can mean your urine is clear even though you are still dehydrated. This is because the body is still catching up on electrolyte losses, such as sodium and potassium (see chapter 5 for more on this), so it removes some water as urine to ensure the sodium level in your blood does not become diluted. When you have replaced the lost water and sodium from sweat, the body's fluid balance will be restored.

Most of the time, you can use water for fluid replacement and food for electrolyte replacement. Sometimes a sports drink can be a rapid way of replacing both together while also getting carbohydrate for energy replacement. This is particularly useful for people who have lost large volumes of sweat, exercised intensely for some hours and have another training session coming up in the next 24 hours or so.

Milk contains electrolytes, fluid, carbohydrate and some protein, so is a great recovery food and fluid all in one. Smoothies with fruit, yoghurt, milk or other similar ingredients help restore all components, and can be an easy way of getting nutrients in when tired.

Soup is perfect for rehydrating, replacing water and electrolytes. Soup generally has a stock base that contains sodium (salt), which helps restore electrolyte levels. We all lose sodium in our sweat. Many foods in our diet provide us with sodium; we just need to balance this with fluid intake.

Having a variety of fluids can aid with rehydration and prevent 'flavour fatigue', which can set in when having sweet drinks all the time. They become unpalatable, prompting us to reduce our fluid intake and increasing the risk of dehydration. This is a concern during endurance events. 'Wet foods' are options that provide variety – think yoghurt, custard, rice pudding and soups.

ALCOHOL AND RECOVERY

In Australia, particularly in team sports, there is a culture of having a few beers after a game of footy or a round of golf, for example. It is important to be aware that alcohol may:

- » slow the restoration of muscle glycogen (stored energy in the muscles)
- » distract the athlete from their feeding regime, which is required in order to replace carbohydrate, protein and other fluids
- » increase blood vessel dilation, which can interfere with healing of any injuries, knocks (bruising) and swelling
- » delay rehydration, due to its diuretic effect.

Consider strategies to delay drinking in cultures where you expect it. For example, you could have coaches address players to discuss the need for recovery prior to drinking alcohol, provide plenty of food to eat, and plenty of non-alcoholic beverages, have areas where alcohol is not allowed, such as change rooms, and have time frames that help delay when the drinking begins.

Consider your recovery goals and safe drinking limits, and recover with food and non-alcoholic fluids first.

THE IMMUNE SYSTEM AND RECOVERY

The body has a stress hormone response to exercise, meaning it increases levels of certain hormones, which makes the immune system more vulnerable to pathogens. Carbohydrate can help protect and reduce the disturbance to the immune system by helping return the hormones to normal levels more quickly. For this reason, it is important to:

- » have adequate carbohydrate stores before exercise
- » ingest carbohydrate during prolonged intense exercise
- » include carbohydrate in your recovery regime.

Having optimal gut health also protects the body from unwanted pathogens, particularly at vulnerable times such as immediately after exercise. There is more information and strategies to maximise protection in chapter 9 (page 93).

BARRIERS TO RECOVERY NUTRITION

There are two key barriers to recovery nutrition: loss of appetite, and unavailability of appropriate recovery food.

LOSS OF APPETITE

In working in men's elite team sport, I have discovered that one of the main reasons for not eating or drinking after exercise is that players are too exhausted at the end of a game. They often feel nauseous, and need to wait a while.

After exercise, moist foods are easier to eat or drink. The loss of fluid during exercise can leave you with a dry mouth, and fatigue can make even chewing too great an effort. Food that can be held in one hand and is portable also works well, as players are often walking around for a cool-down or to talk to friends. Elite athletes also often have commitments with media, coaches, medical staff and family that require them to be moving around.

Foods that I have found to be popular in this situation are:

- chicken wraps or pitas (with a sauce to moisten)
- pasta with a meat sauce
- chicken risotto
- beef or bean burritos
- lean-meat hamburgers
- fruit
- rice pudding
- toast with avocado and Vegemite
- milk smoothies and milk.

AVAILABILITY

The food that is available at a venue can sometimes limit food choices for recovery. For example, is there a canteen with any healthy choices, or just vending machines with poor choices?

If working with a team, what can be delivered to a venue? The venue itself may impose restrictions on food being brought in rather than ordered from on-site catering. I have found this to be a limitation when working with AFL teams. Alternatives such as using external caterers requires research into what can be cooked close to the game's finishing time and delivered in bulk, either hot or cold, to the venue, as well as arranging security clearance so caterers can gain access to the arena. A senior or junior sports team who have had to travel to their game and have a long journey home might benefit from a nutritious choice being delivered to the venue, rather than families grabbing takeaway on the drive home. If setting out early to travel to a venue, having food ready for the team to top up when they arrive can also be a saviour.

If you are going to be at an event for a long period, consider how you will keep your food cool if it requires refrigeration. This may limit the dairy and meat products you can bring, unless you can transport your food in cooler bags and with ice.

Sponsors of events and teams can determine what food and fluid is going to be offered. For example, sports drinks handed out at a fun run will generally be a sponsor's product. Make sure you are aware of what will be offered, and bring your own if that food is not suitable. For elite sports teams, only sponsored product is available in the change rooms for players. This can be difficult if the sponsor's product is not the most appropriate food choice for players, or if more variety is desired. If the athlete doesn't like what is available, this may hinder recovery.

You can see that individual circumstances and goals will determine what your recovery regime should involve in order to optimally fuel you.

HIGH-CARBOHYDRATE RECOVERY FOOD IDEAS

- breads, rolls, pita, dry biscuits
- fruit – fresh, canned or dried
- grains – quinoa, couscous, rice, noodles, pasta, lupins, freekeh
- legumes – chickpeas, baked beans, kidney beans
- milk, yoghurt (also contains protein), custard, rice pudding
- potato, sweet potato, corn
- breakfast cereal, muesli bars (watch for quality)
- sports drinks, fruit juice (consider when these are needed and how much)

PROTEIN FOODS FOR RECOVERY (~10 GRAMS PROTEIN)

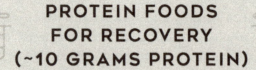

Using the following list as a guide, you can combine various foods to meet your protein needs for recovery.

- milk, 300 ml
- eggs, 2 × 55 g
- yoghurt, 200 g
- quark yoghurt, 110 g
- cheese, 30 g
- cottage cheese, 70 g
- chicken, 40 g cooked
- beef, 35 g cooked
- fish, fresh or canned, 50 g
- soft tofu, 120 g
- cooked lentils, ½ cup
- cooked green peas, 1 cup
- cooked quinoa, 1 cup

CHAPTER 14

Do Nutrition Needs Change with Age?

OLDER ATHLETES

What is classified as an older athlete? Masters athletes in many sports are the ripe young age of 35 to 40 years! I do notice an enormous difference in the nutritional needs of a footy player who is 18 and one who is 30. I wouldn't call the 30-year-old player old; however, in elite sport they are considered the 'older athlete'.

In this chapter we are looking at an older age group than this – around 55+ years, where individual nutritional needs are starting to change. As we age, our quality of health varies, and this can alter people's nutritional needs. It is important to consider chronological age versus biological age. Medications and chronic disease become more prevalent with age, which can affect nutritional recommendations.

Optimal nutrition has a positive impact not only on sporting performance, but also on the risk of chronic disease. By focusing on improving your diet in order to fuel physical activity, you develop a positive mindset about eating, which keeps you motivated. I have found that 'eating like an athlete', focusing on what you can eat rather than what you can't, is a real winner, particularly with people aged over 60 of varying activity levels.

In my private practice I am seeing more people aged in their late forties either taking up sport or continuing with it and being competitive, striving for PBs (personal bests), and ticking off items on their bucket list such as completing a half or full marathon, a hike or a triathlon. Adequate nutrition to support this is essential. For some of these individuals, it is the first time they have actually looked at how their diet relates to performance.

I have a male client around the age of 55 who loves going to the gym. He has two goals: one is to lift heavier weights, and the other is to minimise the body fat that has been creeping up around his abdominal area. This combination of goals has him thinking about what he can eat to benefit his performance and health, rather than just focusing on his abdomen and disease prevention. He thinks of foods to eat pre- and post-gym.

Pre-gym, he might eat a yoghurt and some nuts in the afternoon while at his desk, and then when he gets home, his motivation means he prepares a dinner that will aid his recovery, rather than grabbing whatever first comes to hand. He thinks about a protein source, whether it be fish, lean meat or eggs, vegetables for antioxidants to aid recovery, and potato for some carbohydrate to ensure he has enough energy for the next day's session. This might not be fancy, but he is getting the balance he needs. This 'eating like an athlete' mentality will improve his gym performance, which is important to him, and his overall health will also benefit.

ENERGY NEEDS OF THE OLDER ATHLETE

People often blame weight gain in later life on a reduction in their metabolism due to age. This is partly true. Your basal metabolism is the rate at which your body burns energy at rest. As we age, we lose muscle mass. Because muscle tissue burns more energy than fat tissue, this means your metabolism does reduce somewhat. With a lower metabolism, you need less energy, and any excess energy is stored as body fat. Being less active as you age can be a contributing factor to weight gain, and can also result in further loss of muscle mass. Keep moving, fuel yourself to do so, and make sure you're getting enough protein!

MICRONUTRIENT NEEDS OF THE OLDER ATHLETE

Even if your energy needs have reduced, your general nutrient needs, particularly your micronutrient (vitamins and minerals) and protein needs, won't have. In fact, some nutrients are needed in larger amounts as we get older, such as calcium for women in peri-menopause (the transition that begins several years prior to menopause, usually in a woman's forties, when the ovaries start to make less oestrogen) and for women post-menopause (when the ovaries stop releasing eggs). It is difficult to set exact targets due to the big difference in the rate of ageing and the variety of exercise undertaken (from a walking group to marathon). Restricting your energy intake due to a focus on weight loss can be detrimental, as this can mean you don't take in enough food to fulfil your micronutrient needs. Try to focus on health more than on weight.

We know that changes occur with ageing. Choosing nutrient-dense foods is critical in order to support these changes. Nutrient-dense foods are those that are packed with nutritional value, such as vitamins, minerals, dietary fibre and protein.

Calcium

Calcium is one of the minerals we need in greater amounts. As we age, our bone density decreases (this occurs in women from around 45 years of age and in men from around 50 years of age), so we need to continually top up our calcium stores to delay this loss. Bones are active tissue, meaning they continually require minerals and protein to maintain strength.

We can slow the decline by eating calcium-containing foods and doing weight-bearing exercise. If you already have low bone density (e.g. osteoporosis, osteopenia) then be cautious when exercising, as your risk of fractures, including stress fractures, will be greater. This is particularly critical for those playing a contact sport.

Dairy foods are a rich source of easily absorbed calcium. You can obtain your recommended daily intake of calcium by including 3–4 serves of dairy foods per day. A serve could be a glass of milk (250 ml), a tub of yoghurt (200 g), a slice of cheese (40 g). Low-fat dairy options contain similar levels of calcium to full-fat versions.

It is not essential to obtain your calcium from dairy; some people prefer plant sources. Plant foods, although much lower in calcium, are still valuable sources of calcium, particularly for vegan athletes. A combination of calcium-containing foods is what most people aim for, giving variety to their overall diet.

NUTRIENT REFERENCE VALUES FOR CALCIUM – AUSTRALIAN RECOMMENDED DIETARY INTAKE	
AGE	RDI
Men	
19–30 years	1000 mg/day
31–50 years	1000 mg/day
51–70 years	1000 mg/day
>70 years	1300 mg/day
Women	
19–30 years	1000 mg/day
31–50 years	1000 mg/day
51–70 years	1300 mg/day
>70 years	1300 mg/day

SOURCES OF CALCIUM

Here are some examples of calcium-containing foods and the quantities needed to obtain one serve (~330 mg) of calcium:

- 250-millilitre glass of milk
- 200-gram tub yoghurt
- 40 grams cheese (2 slices)
- 100 grams tofu
- 250-millilitres soy drink (fortified, added calcium)
- 90-gram can sardines
- 12 dried figs
- 2 cups cooked silverbeet (or similar greens)
- 600 grams soy beans, canned
- 100 grams almonds.

Try the following ideas to boost your calcium intake:

- Eat the bones of canned salmon or sardines, as they are rich in calcium.
- Add yoghurt to soups or salads.
- Add milk or skim milk powder to soups or casseroles.
- Try soy-based products, such as soy milk with added calcium, and tofu.
- Include broccoli, mustard cabbage, bok choy, silverbeet, cucumber, celery and chickpeas in your diet, as they all contain some calcium.
- Eat almonds, dried figs and dried apricots (remember, dried fruit is a concentrated form of sugar).
- Look for products fortified with calcium, such as some breakfast cereals.

Vitamin D

Vitamin D is also important for bone health. The skin's ability to convert and use sunlight to initiate the vitamin D activation process is diminished with age, meaning more vitamin D is needed.

It is important to have your vitamin D levels checked, particularly if you are living and training mostly indoors, or if you cover up to protect from the sun most of the time. In some cases, a calcium and vitamin D supplement might be needed.

Most of our vitamin D comes from exposure to the sun; however, oily fish, liver, eggs, cheese, and mushrooms that have been exposed to UV light or that you sit on your windowsill all contain some vitamin D (one-hundred grams of mushrooms exposed to an hour of winter sunlight will develop your vitamin D needs for the day). How much sunlight you need will depend on where you live and your skin type. Refer to the Cancer Council of Australia's recommendations for skin exposure times.

Iron

The recommended daily intake for iron is lower for adults aged over 50, as iron requirements reduce slightly with ageing. For example, after women go through menopause, the monthly menstruation that can result in iron loss stops. However, athletes require more iron than non-athletes, therefore eating adequate iron is still essential, particularly for endurance athletes. A blood test can measure iron levels if you are concerned.

Vitamin C

Vitamin C is essential for:

» your immune system – more vitamin C is needed if you have an illness. For example, vitamin C can help reduce the symptoms and duration of the common cold.

» collagen formation – collagen is the structural material of bones, muscles and skin

» skin integrity and wound healing – skin becomes thinner as you age, and can tear more easily.

Wounds increase your requirement for vitamin C. In 2016 in a Sydney hospital study, some patients with diabetes who had wounds were found to be suffering from scurvy, generally known as the disease early sailors died from due to the lack of vitamin C in their diet. The patients' wounds were not healing due to inadequate vitamin C.

Ageing and exercise cause increased oxidative stress, which increases vitamin C requirements. Eating two pieces of fresh fruit daily will generally give you adequate vitamin C, but if your body is healing this need will increase, and some individuals may benefit from supplementation. Raw vegetables (for instance capsicum), or vegetables that have been lightly cooked (for instance broccoli), are rich sources of vitamin C.

If you are exercising at high intensity, one or two extra serves of high vitamin C-containing foods could help boost your compromised immune system.

Zinc

The RDI for zinc is the same for the older population as it is for the younger, unless illness strikes or repair is required. Zinc is involved in tissue repair and immune function. Older athletes are more susceptible to injury, and therefore zinc is very important. As we age, it is important that we continue to eat zinc-rich foods. Meat, seafood, wholegrains, legumes and nuts are all valuable sources of zinc. Like iron, zinc is best absorbed from animal products. If you take calcium or iron supplements with meals, be aware that they will reduce the absorption of zinc, so it is best to take them at separate times.

PROTEIN NEEDS OF THE OLDER ATHLETE

As we age, muscle wasting (sarcopenia) occurs, which results in a loss of strength and possibly function. This is due to protein synthesis impairment of the ageing skeletal muscle. To help reduce muscle wasting, we need to ensure there is sufficient protein in our diet.

It is important to spread protein intake out over the day. This gives the most benefit. It is thought that our body uses protein less efficiently as we age, meaning we require more in order to achieve the same effect.

Having a protein and carbohydrate-containing snack close to finishing exercise (within 30–60 minutes) seems to be particularly important for older athletes – it stimulates muscle building, rather than breaking down.

The same principles apply to older athletes as to other age groups, in that individuals engaging in strength training and power sports may require more protein. Requirements will, of course, be individual and vary, but most people will require between 1.5 and 2 grams of protein per kilogram of body weight, depending on their age, health and activity level. Research from the University of Birmingham suggests that an athlete over the age of 80 years may benefit from a protein intake of 2+ grams per kilogram of body weight. Eating some protein 4–5 times per day in meals or snacks may be beneficial in order to maintain muscle mass.

Protein intake sometimes reduces with age, due to a reduction in the volume of food eaten. Declines in dental health can also result in reduced meat intake due to difficulty with chewing – a good reason those dreaded six-monthly dental checks are so important. If chewing meat is an issue, soft, moist meats and fish, eggs, tofu and dairy can be good alternative protein sources. Having a glass of warm milk before bed to maximise overnight synthesis and repair is also a good idea.

PHYSIOLOGICAL CHANGES IN THE OLDER ATHLETE

Bodily functions change as we age, and at varying rates. For example, older individuals often experience a decrease in thirst. Kidney function also reduces with age, with kidneys losing fluid that they would once have reabsorbed. Older athletes need to monitor fluid intake closely, and should not rely on just thirst as an indicator of hydration status. Other indicators, such as frequency of urination, become very important (see chapter 5 for more on hydration).

The thermoregulatory (temperature) response also deteriorates as we age. This is due to changes in the functioning of the cardiovascular system. Blood output from the heart reduces, meaning less blood flow goes to the skin, where heat is normally lost, resulting in an increased risk of heat stress.

BLOOD SUGAR LEVELS OF THE OLDER ATHLETE

As we age, it is important to monitor health markers such as blood sugar levels. This will often be done annually, during a general check by your general practitioner (GP). If you find that your blood sugar levels are creeping up, a few modifications to your diet might help keep them in control, avoiding health complications and still allowing you to be active. This can be particularly relevant if you have a large carbohydrate requirement due to a lot of aerobic activity – for example, endurance events, long bike rides, walks or even hikes. Knowing how much carbohydrate you need, what type and how to spread it out over the day is important.

An older couple I once worked with had started swimming each morning. The wife had diabetes to contend with, so I recommended low-GI carbohydrates to fuel her for the swim and for day-to-day life. Her healthy breakfast of a bowl of oats combined with natural yoghurt and milk for more protein, along with a sprinkle of seeds and nuts, worked perfectly. She eats until she is comfortable and checks her blood sugar level 2 hours later. The volume of breakfast can be increased or reduced as needed, and the carbohydrate in the following meal can be adjusted based on how she is feeling and her blood glucose reading.

Changes that may improve high blood sugar levels include:

- » reducing the carbohydrate load at some meals
- » eating more wholegrain cereals
- » eating more vegetables
- » swapping foods around to different times
- » including some protein and healthy fats at each meal and snack, such as yoghurt or nuts with fruit, or cheese on a cracker rather than just the cracker on its own.

BOWEL HEALTH IN OLDER ATHLETES

Another issue that arises as we age is bowel health. Your bowel relies on peristaltic motion to push things along – a bit like squeezing the toothpaste down the tube, and as ageing occurs this muscular action can become weaker.

The neurological signals between the brain and the gut can also change as we age, and some medications can affect bowel regularity. Irregular or haphazard bowel motions can be daunting. If they are keeping you from being active, seek medical advice to find out what can be done to help you remain active. Some dietary changes and other interventions may assist.

If bowels become less regular and constipation is an issue, an increase in dietary fibre might be beneficial. It is important to include a variety of fibres in the diet, such as fruit, vegetables, lentils, legumes and a variety of whole grains (not all wheat-based). Maximising gut bacteria (these can also reduce with age, and can be affected by medications) and drinking plenty of fluid are also important for optimal bowel function.

Keep up your exercise so you don't miss out on the fun, socialising, fitness, feel-good hormones and health benefits. You may need to alter your nutritional intake as you grow older. Just remember, your needs are yours – everyone is individual, and this becomes even more evident as we age.

YOUNGER ATHLETES

The basic principles of sports nutrition recommended for adults also apply to children and adolescents, but there are some unique periods, particularly during growth spurts, when the younger athlete's nutritional needs increase. Here, when we talk about the younger athlete, we are referring to those aged between 6 and 18 years.

The younger years are a great time to start developing healthy eating habits, and participation in sport can help encourage young athletes to take an interest in the topic. Many aspire to compete at an elite level, like their heroes, and are motivated to do their best to get there. Even those who don't aspire to become elite are generally keen to perform at their best, and to understand how food can help them do this.

Eating like an athlete is a positive approach, and one that can help teach young people about the food that will fuel their body and help them grow. General health messages such as those relating to heart health and cancer prevention are also important, but it can be hard for children to be motivated about eating well in order to prevent a disease that might be thirty or more years down the track.

I have worked with primary and secondary school children who are serious swimmers, tennis players and footballers. They show an interest in learning about what to pack in their lunch box to fuel them for after-school training, what to have for dinner for recovery and what to take on competition day to give them an edge. Their passion for their sport is what fuels their interest.

The following is an overview of some things to look out for in younger athletes.

OVERHEATING AND FLUID INTAKE

Their smaller body volume means young people can dehydrate and overheat more rapidly. Drinking extra fluid in hot environments is essential. Water is best most of the time, but if they are exercising intensely in hot conditions for 60 minutes or more, something flavoured and containing electrolytes (e.g. oral rehydration fluids, milk, sports drinks, fruit juice) might be needed. Flavour can encourage drinking, helping to ensure sufficient intake. This should be monitored on an individual basis. Avoid sipping on sugar-containing flavoured drinks for long periods, as this is bad for dental health.

ENERGY NEEDS

Young athletes will need extra energy during growth spurts and periods of high training loads. It is important that the young athlete listens to their body and their hunger, and understands that sometimes they will need to eat more, and at other times less. Eating nutritious snacks becomes important, as often young people become full at mealtimes before they have met their needs, so snacks can be the top-up. It is important to be mindful of dental health, however. Like for any age group, sweet, sticky foods and drinks should be kept to a minimum.

Children are usually good at knowing when they are full and when they are hungry. As adults, we need to trust this so they don't lose this awareness. Many adults are not good at listening to their own hunger and fullness cues.

I remember a client who was concerned that her primary-school-aged daughter's diet was not as nutritious as it could be, and feared that she was overweight. Soft drink was a regular part of the family diet, so I suggested keeping it for special occasions and not having it as a regular fridge item in the home. I discouraged talk about dieting and weight, and suggested the family focus on choosing foods for feeling fit and healthy and looking after their bodies, including their teeth. On the return visit the client complained, 'She has not been following your suggestions.'

I thought this was unfair on such a young girl. Soft drink was still being kept in the fridge at home. It is hard to expect an adult to break a habit, let alone a child. Anyone attempting to make long-term change needs to be supported by the people around them. Young athletes sometimes find this difficult when other family members are not athletes and the food at home is not what they need to optimally fuel them. I encourage parents to look at the whole household, including themselves. Everyone can benefit from eating like an athlete – modifying volumes and stocking the fridge and cupboards with nutritious, tasty foods. Don't focus on weight, focus on fuelling a healthy body and being active.

IRON AND THE YOUNG ATHLETE

Iron requirements increase at the age of 14 years for both boys and girls; however, this increase is greater in girls, because they generally start to menstruate around this age. Boys aged 14–18 years need around 11 mg of iron per day; girls aged 14–18 years need 15 mg per day. Women have greater iron requirements than men until they reach menopause at around the age of 50.

It is also important to keep a careful eye on iron levels if a young athlete decides to follow a vegetarian or vegan diet, or chooses not to eat red meat. Extra legumes, lentils, green leafy vegetables and eggs, if not following a vegan diet, should be included.

If a young athlete shows signs of greater fatigue than usual, this may be due to low iron levels. These can be checked by talking to the GP and having a blood test. Fatigue can be due to many things, however – low iron is just one of them.

GET IN THE KITCHEN YOUNG

One of the most valuable things I can suggest a young person should do is to learn how to prepare food for themselves. Some basic cooking skills will go a long way in ensuring healthy food choices, enabling young people to come home from school and make scrambled eggs, cook a basic dinner of meat and vegetables, or throw together a pasta dish. The athletes I have worked with who started cooking while still living at home were so much better prepared when they then lived on their own. They shop for food confidently and can prepare a basic meal without stress, meeting their nutritional needs and giving them the fuel they need to train at their best. Those who haven't developed the basic skills tend to struggle, and cooking becomes a chore at the end of a long day.

Learning how to chop up vegetables, cook pasta and rice, grill meats and make a basic pasta sauce can get them a long way. One country boy who had a few cooking skills attended one of our AFL club cooking sessions, where he perfected his beef and vegetable risotto bake. It became his signature dish, and he cooked it for his host family weekly!

SECTION 3
STRATEGIES FOR HEALTHY EATING

CHAPTER 15
Making Lifestyle Changes

What changes could you make to your lifestyle to improve your nutrition in order to achieve optimal sporting performance and health? How can you make your environment elite? This is something I encourage professional athletes to think about. They have the advantage of an elite training environment, but how does the rest of their lifestyle match up?

FOOD IN YOUR WORKPLACE

Most of us are not professional athletes, so our workplace is not generally set up to support our nutrition goals. Due to the many hours we spend at work, the food we consume there has a substantial impact on our overall diet.

Some workplaces provide breakfast options such as cereal, milk, fruit and bread (most elite sports teams certainly do), which can help if you have trained early in the morning or are running late for work. If your workplace doesn't supply these things, think about bringing in a stock of your own, or encourage them to.

SUGGESTIONS FOR A NUTRITIOUS WORKPLACE

Some workplace initiatives that could boost employees' health include:

» supplying fresh fruit, nuts, yoghurt, wholegrain dry biscuits, cheese, eggs and oats to make breakfast, instead of a tin of sweet biscuits

- » encouraging group walking at lunchtime or after work, and holding walking meetings to support an overall health philosophy. Sometimes we train for an hour and then sit for the rest of the day. We need incidental exercise, too.
- » providing information about healthy lunch options that are available to purchase nearby, and negotiating a discount for workers on the healthy meal choice of the day
- » having work celebrations and morning teas that extend beyond cake or a huge muffin (which is really just a big piece of cake), offering healthier options such as tasty, smaller muffins (made with ingredients such as wholemeal flour, rolled oats, nuts, fruit, chia seeds and vegetables for savoury options), a fresh fruit platter, fresh sandwiches, wraps, salads, soups, rice paper rolls, nuts, seeds, dried fruit or yoghurt tubs, with a few small, decadent cakes occasionally. Healthy snacks such as these are perfect pre-training options for people who will be active in the afternoon, or as recovery foods for those who exercise at lunchtime.
- » organising soup, salad or curry days, where a group of people are rostered on to bring in a meal once a month to share. This can be a fun social activity that encourages healthy eating.
- » celebrating all the birthdays in a month together on one day, rather than having a cake every second day, and including other choices in addition to cake.

Wellness goes a long way towards increasing overall productivity and reducing sick days, so it's well worth the investment.

HEALTHY EATING IN A SPORTING CLUB

It is encouraging to see people being active and social within sporting clubs, but the nutritional value of the food provided by some establishments could definitely be improved. It's not about having everything perfect, it's about providing options, and making it easy for people to make healthy choices in order to support the great work of being active.

What does your club supply? Do they have a canteen? Often this is run by volunteers, so the workload needs to be kept to a minimum. Frozen food that can be purchased in bulk is appealing, because it is quick, produces minimal waste and can be kept on site until needed. Fresh ingredients require planning and preparation, and unfortunately sometimes there is waste. However, they also come with health benefits, so it is worth motivating people to put in the effort.

Planning to include fresh ingredients requires working out approximately how many servings are likely to be sold, and ordering some healthier packaged items (e.g. soups, ravioli, corn on the cob, steamed instead of fried dumplings or dim sims), 100 per cent fruit icy poles, and bottles of sparkling and plain water. Discounts or sponsorship might be negotiated by talking with local food suppliers such as bakers, greengrocers and supermarkets.

The location of food items can also influence what people buy. Have the fresh food presented in an appealing manner that is easily visible. For example, in warmer weather, offer foods such as:

- » freshly cut watermelon ready to go
- » tubs of yoghurt on ice
- » rice paper rolls
- » chocolate-dipped frozen bananas.

And in the cooler weather, try things like:

- » hot soup
- » corn on the cob
- » roast beef rolls
- » toasted sandwiches.

There are plenty of appealing ideas. Get members involved in deciding what will be available, as ownership is the key to success.

Does the club provide meals at functions, after training or at competitions? Having a basic policy around what food and fluids are served avoids having to make these decisions each time an event arises. It could cover the canteen as well. For example, the policy may consider not serving deep-fried food or soft drink. There may be guidelines around what types of fluid will be provided and when. Water may be the main drink, for example, with sports drink or cordial being offered at certain times, such as during competition or when the weather is over 30° Celsius. Soft drink may only be available at club celebratory dinners.

I don't believe lollies should be the go-to at half time. What happened to half-time oranges? They are perfect, easy to prepare, economical and provide fluid, some sugar and electrolytes. Any cut-up fruit would be great. If the day is long, rolls, sandwiches, plain muesli bars (even though they're not great for your teeth), soup, slices of cheese, yoghurt and hard-boiled eggs are all fairly easy, healthy choices for adults and children to snack on. These are just suggestions, of course. Each club will have its own needs, and an accredited sports dietitian could help develop a suitable policy.

Have plenty of water available, preferably supplied free of charge in jugs, bubblers and easily accessible taps, as well as bottles to purchase if desired. In Aussie Rules, Rugby League and other sporting codes, it might also be suitable to provide sports drinks in limited amounts around match time.

Alcohol is always a tricky issue at sporting clubs. Have a variety of non-alcoholic drinks available, both for those who are not drinking alcohol and to provide alternatives to those who are. Help people understand why it is important to limit alcohol and provide other choices. It is not about being a wet blanket, it is facilitating the club to provide a supportive environment, making healthy choices the easy choices.

SOCIAL MEDIA'S INFLUENCE ON HEALTH

There is a lot of advice out there on social media regarding food and nutrition. Choose what you read and who you follow wisely. There are plenty of 'perfect people' online – models, entertainers, sports heroes – who appear to be living 'perfect lives'. Remember, they are showcasing their highlights when at their best. This is so important to remember from a body image perspective and as a person who is fitting in both work and exercise. Some of the people you follow are elite athletes – remember, being fit and healthy is their job, they work at it all day long. Keep it in perspective.

Do you find yourself aspiring to a body shape or size that is unachievable, and maybe unnecessary (more muscles, thinner, curves in different places)? Do you feel that you should cook a perfectly plated and nutritionally balanced meal every night? Catch yourself if you are doing this, and make sure you're not being too hard on yourself – show self-compassion. Follow and connect with what inspires you, rather than makes you feel guilty. Avoid those who bring you down and make you feel inadequate. Unfollow anyone whose posts prompt you to talk negatively to yourself. Stick with those who inspire you and make you feel good. Read stories that give you practical strategies you can implement, that are realistic and relevant, and that bring a smile to your face.

GETTING THE HOUSEHOLD ON BOARD

FUSSY EATERS – BIG AND SMALL

What you want to eat and what others in your household want to eat don't always align. Let's have a look at ways you can make the household meals work for you.

» Be a good role model — eat a balanced variety and a decent amount of nutritious foods and drinks, so others can follow your lead.
» Young children are often tired at the end of the day. If they don't eat their dinner it may not be because they don't like it – they could just be too tired for chewing, trying new foods and eating in general. Consider what time you have your meals, and what form they take. Kids often like to eat with their hands. Give them vegetables that can be picked up – peas, beans, carrot, capsicum, cucumber sticks, cherry tomatoes or corn on the cob, for example.
» Make homemade healthier versions of some favourite takeaway foods, rather than cutting them out altogether. For example, hamburgers, meatballs, souvlaki, kebabs, pizza, fish and chips, chicken strips, jacket potatoes, rice paper rolls, burritos, toasted sandwiches and wraps. Have fun by getting everyone in the kitchen to choose their own toppings and additions to these foods.

» Spread the load, and encourage everyone in the household to develop cooking skills and a love of cooking. That way one person isn't burdened with the load of cooking and menu-planning.
» Let everyone have input into the food that's kept in the fridge and pantry, and into deciding the weekly dinner menu. If people feel ownership, they will participate.

TRYING NEW FOODS

In order to like a new food, you've got to try it around ten times. A big part of what makes up your sense of taste is smell. If a smell is foreign to you, or you don't like the smell of a food when it's cooking, then you've already decided that you're not going to like it. The same goes for sight. If a food doesn't look appetising, you've already decided you won't like it. Encourage yourself and others to get past this. The same goes for texture. If this is unfamiliar, again, you may find yourself saying you don't like the food.

Over ten tastings you'll gradually get used to the smell, appearance, texture and taste of a food, which is when you'll probably like it. When I'm presenting a group talk I often challenge the audience to think of a fruit or vegetable that is nutritious and that they wish they enjoyed, and to try it on ten different occasions. I can just about guarantee they will like it by the tenth go.

When I introduce new foods to the Hawthorn football team I am usually present to explain what the food is and why it is beneficial to performance. If the players can see some benefit, they will usually have a go. The benefits might include the food being quick and easy to eat, requiring minimal preparation, being available in their local supermarket and reasonably priced, tasting pretty good and having a nutritional benefit. All these factors combine to determine whether it will become a new addition to their diet. For example, I once introduced them to a range of ready-made legume salads. They don't look all that appealing, but their protein, carbohydrate, dietary fibre and vitamin content makes them a perfect addition to a meal or as a post-training snack. They come in a single-serve, easy-to-open container.

I encourage my brother, who has Down syndrome, to eat fruit. When I asked him why he wasn't eating passionfruit, he said, 'too seedy'. I asked about watermelon and he said, 'too watery'. It was the textures that weren't appealing to him. If he keeps trying them over a few weeks he might change his mind as familiarity increases, but as it's not a priority to him, and I'm not around to offer them regularly, he still doesn't like them.

I used to dislike the taste of mango and avocado. I thought mangos smelt like kerosene and avocados like bad eggs, so I refused to try them. Later, I realised that both were easy foods to mash and feed to my children when they were babies. I did it often enough that I grew to like the smell, the texture (which I now think of as velvety) and the taste. I love them both now! That was at 30 years of age – you're never too old to try a new food and increase your repertoire.

When introducing a new food, it's best to offer a small amount, along with other foods that you know the people in your household like. Don't make too much fuss about the new food – you don't want mealtimes to become a battle zone. Simply serve up a small amount on the plate. Even if they don't eat it at first, gradually they will become more familiar with the look and smell, and will soon decide to try it.

When my daughter was about three years old she used to take the peas and beans individually off her plate and put them on the table. We made a rule that they had to stay on the plate, even if she didn't eat them. Eventually she started trying them, and experimenting – including one time when she put a pea up her nose!

I have had many parents of young athletes bring their children to see me because they are fussy eaters. It is more difficult to meet their energy and protein requirements if they will only eat a narrow range of foods. This limited range means they often make poor nutritional food choices, particularly when choosing snacks. The greater the variety of food, the greater the variety of vitamins, minerals and antioxidants in their diet.

SUPPORT AROUND YOU

To help you continue your healthy eating habits long term, look for support. It's much easier to maintain long-term habits when the people you spend time with are on the same or a similar journey, or at least understand the one you are on. It can be easy for others to sabotage your good intentions, not deliberately, but because they are not ready to change themselves. If others aren't on the same journey, that's okay, but let them know your intentions and ask for their support. For example, if you're trying to give up soft drink but it's always in the fridge at home and on the table during meals, it'll be near impossible to break the habit. It's much easier if it's not there, or is limited.

I find that athletes living together usually succeed with optimal nutrition if at least one of them is committed to good nutrition practices and can lead the others in the right direction, particularly with cooking and eating at home.

Having influencers on board in your household, workplace, sporting club (including coaches) and even among your friends and extended family will make a difference to driving nutrition messages and making positive change.

LOOK BEYOND WEIGHT LOSS AND DIETS

Clients often come to see me because they were told by a doctor, other health professional or coach that they need to lose weight to improve their health and/or performance. Many have diabetes, high blood pressure and/or high cholesterol, and have dieted for many years without success, leaving them feeling deflated and defeated. What they need is a new strategy and focus, not another new fad dieting regime.

Most athletes are not what would be considered overweight in the general population. The definition of overweight in sport, however, depends on the sport, and often on someone's opinion. This can put an awful lot of pressure on the athlete – often unfairly and unnecessarily.

Modifying body composition (e.g. increasing muscle, losing body fat) may aid some sporting performances for some people, but it is not a change that must happen before performance improves, nor is it a guarantee that it will. Long-term restrictive dieting is certainly not an ingredient for success – it is mentally, emotionally and sometimes physically draining. The focus on dietary intake should be a positive one, looking at aspects such as fuelling the body for training sessions and competitions, minimising the risk of illness, focusing on general health needs and, of course, on enjoyment.

Occasionally, an athlete may be in a situation where weight loss is required, such as in weight category sports where the athlete is over the required weight range. The best strategy is to plan for the change in body composition well in advance so a restrictive diet is not required, and certainly not needed long term.

Removing the constant focus on weight loss may result in weight reduction or stabilisation of weight anyway, along with health improvements, without the guilt that fad dieting cycles drive.

Exercise to improve your health, and eat like an athlete, even if you don't consider yourself one. Everyone can be an athlete at their own level. This is a far more positive way to look at your food intake than dieting or focusing on losing weight. Remove the weight-loss focus and look at which foods will fuel you for your life. Rather than using scales, measure improvements with health markers and performance, such as:

- » improvements in blood glucose, blood pressure, blood cholesterol, liver function, kidney function, stress hormone levels
- » increased bone density
- » a reduced need for medications due to improved health
- » improved energy levels
- » increasing strength (increasing muscle)
- » increasing endurance (walking or cycling further, making it through eighteen holes of golf easily, not nine).

Being able to participate in activities you once couldn't is encouraging, and can improve your quality of life.

At the beginning of 2016 an older couple came to see me, having been referred by their GP. Although her husband came along too, the wife was technically the client. She was a perfect example of someone who has had weight loss as her focus and has struggled with it unsuccessfully for years. They had started swimming, which was very important for the wife's arthritis. I approached our consultation by suggesting that we look at her diet as 'eating like an athlete'. They started swimming at 5.30 am on weekdays. We began to approach her eating from the perspective of how it could benefit her health, focusing on her arthritis and improving her energy levels.

They began to consider breakfast as recovery food post-swimming. They planned lunch by focusing on what they would include (such as extra vegetables, protein and calcium), rather than what they would remove. Protein was a focus for muscle maintenance, along with healthy fats (including extra virgin olive oil and omega 3 fatty acids in fish) and plenty of vegetables for anti-inflammatory benefits to help with the woman's arthritis.

Her energy levels increased dramatically as a result of her improved fitness and the change in her food choices. Her blood pressure and blood glucose levels were reduced, her bowel motions became more regular and the pressure of dieting had gone. She learnt to eat more mindfully, listen to her appetite and body signals, and remove the guilt connected with eating, improving her relationship with and her enjoyment of food.

At first, her husband swam only one lap, but he progressed over time, eventually swimming up to sixteen laps. What an endurance improvement! On one visit the husband was so pleased with his own health progress that he described their visits as a 'two for one deal'.

It doesn't matter what age you are, eating to fuel your activity and benefit your health is important!

CHANGE YOUR THINKING

I often hear people say 'I am going to give up chocolate or sugar ...' As a long-term goal, this is unrealistic. Even for gold medal–winning performances it is unnecessary. Rather than saying you will never eat a food again, think of strategies that will help you incorporate it into your diet in an amount you feel comfortable with. You don't need to give up a food, you just need to be aware of how much, when, and what you're are eating, and the quantities that will nourish your body best. Here are some strategies:

- **Forget the scales**: Throw the idea of dieting out the window, and maybe the scales, too (just make sure no-one is standing outside the window when you do it). Restrictive, fad diets don't work long term, otherwise we wouldn't be constantly inventing new ones. They can make your life miserable, focusing on what you can't have. Changes to your diet may be needed, but being overly restrictive and following unsustainable fad diets is not the way to make them.

- **Engage selectively with media**: Steer clear of magazines, online articles, TV shows and social media accounts that talk about and promote unrealistic diets and 'perfect' bodies that don't suit you.

- **Remove clothes**: Remove any clothes that don't fit from your wardrobe. If you're not ready to ditch them, pack them up into a suitcase or put them in a part of your wardrobe you don't see every day.

- **Be positive**: No matter what age or stage you are at, think of yourself as an athlete wanting to perform at your best in whatever you are doing. This sets a positive mindset, rather than one of poor health or negativity. Feed your body the foods it needs to perform at its best. It doesn't matter if you start with a walk around the block or you're running a marathon, we are all competing in this event called 'living life to the fullest'.

- **Enjoy food**: Make time for eating. Sit, relax, taste and savour your food. Treats are important too – have them at a time when you can savour the taste, not when you're rushing or starving (these are the times you're likely to overeat).

WHAT IF I NEED TO KNOW MY WEIGHT OR SKINFOLD MEASUREMENTS?

Although I've said to throw away the scales and stop weighing yourself, some athletes do need to know their weight at certain times. A lightweight rower, a competitor in category weight boxing, most elite athletes and the AFL players I work with all monitor their weight to some extent. They may need to be heavier so they can physically compete, or they may need to be lighter to reduce the amount of weight they're putting on an injured knee or ankle, or to help with endurance in long-distance running. They may also weigh themselves to look at fluid losses. The weight focus is very different in these cases. It is not about dieting. Yes, changes may need to be made to the athlete's dietary intake, but weight reduction is not the sole focus. It is also generally planned and gradual, and is sometimes a short-term goal, such as for a weigh-in before a boxing fight.

Measuring body fat levels by taking skinfold measurements using calipers can be daunting. When trying to reduce an athlete's skinfold measurements with the aim of reducing body fat levels, I am very careful about avoiding the dieting mentality. The focus is on proportions of food, such as increasing and decreasing carbohydrate intake, the timing of food around training to fuel sessions and how this can be modified at other times to achieve desired results. There are numerous strategies, but they all primarily focus on what you can eat, rather than on what you can't.

HOW TO MAKE YOUR DIET ELITE WITHOUT DIETING

Here are a few tips I would suggest:

» Upgrade from a low-fibre, high-sugar cereal to something with less added sugar and more dietary fibre (e.g. around 6 grams of fibre per 100 grams), and then move on to one with 8 or more grams of dietary fibre per 100 grams as a guide. Also look for a variety of fibre types.

» Swap out the habitual store-bought sweet biscuits for a handful of fresh nuts – the taste alone will entice you.

» Instead of potato chips, enjoy homemade popcorn cooked in extra virgin olive oil, sprinkled with chilli flakes and a small amount of salt.

» Try reducing nightly ice cream to once or twice per week, and have yoghurt with fresh fruit and nuts on the other nights to add extra nutrients.

» Swap afternoon or after-sport lollies with fruit (e.g. fruit platter, fruit salad, punnet of berries, canned fruit, dried fruit) – this still provides some sugar but with the added benefit of nutrients and dietary fibre.

» Swap snack pack dry biscuits with cream cheese–based dips for cut-up vegetables (red capsicum, carrot, celery, snow peas, mushrooms) or oven-baked pita bread (topped with olive oil and herbs) with natural yoghurt, salsa, or beetroot or hummus-based dips.

» Butter or margarine on white toast could swapped for extra virgin olive oil, a slice of cheese, avocado (great with Vegemite), ricotta, quark or cottage cheese (great with a little jam or honey on top), on wholegrain or sourdough rye toast.

- » Replace blended vegetable oils with extra virgin olive oil.
- » Swap soft drink for a glass of soda water, sparkling water, natural mineral water or milk.
- » Consider replacing takeaway deep-fried fish and chips with grilled fish, a few less chips and a salad. It could be home-cooked fish done on the barbecue or in the oven with baked chips (straight from the freezer if need be) or crusty bread and salad. You will feel so much lighter!

PLANNING FOR CHANGE

To make changes, we need goals and strategies. I like S.M.A.R.T goals – specific, measurable, attainable, realistic and time-based. If your goal is to prepare and eat food at home more often, what strategies will you need to use to make this happen, and how will you measure your success? Set realistic goals. You may need to start more gently with a short-term goal, and work up to your ultimate goal.

For example, your goal might be 'I will eat at home six out of seven nights, and take my lunch to work four out of five days.' My strategies to achieve this would include:

- » Identifying what's going on in the household for the week so the menu can be planned. When is everyone home? What activities occur around dinner time? Who will be home when?
- » Prepare a shopping list and keep it on my phone.
- » Choose a convenient time to shop, and mark it in my diary.
- » Cook extra of our meal on Sunday night to have during the week, and also cook an extra dish to freeze.
- » On Friday night when everyone is tired, have a quick meal, such as homemade hamburgers bought from the butcher, with everyone adding their own toppings.

- » Use quick meal ideas for after work and late training finishes, such as stir-fried frozen vegetables with chicken strips, and ask one of the children to cut up the chicken and marinate it if home early.
- » For a homemade lunch, make a sandwich the night before, and if there are school lunches to make prepare them at the same time (children or others can help so this is less of a chore).
- » Consider when I will be training and what extra snacks I'll need to have ready.
- » Plan what day/night my competition or game is and what food I like to have before and after that.
- » Make a list of what to do instead of eating when I'm stressed or bored, such as listen to music, buy myself flowers, do something physical, kick the footy, visit or phone a friend, take time for a bath, go away for a night or afternoon, go for a walk in a favourite place, or eat my favourite fruit (and make sure the fridge is stocked with this).

IDENTIFY BARRIERS TO MAKING CHANGE

I work with a delightful couple who come and see me for dietary advice. They both work long days – as a manager in a busy hospital and a school principal – and were struggling to regularly prepare meals. The husband already had his lunch preparation down pat, so I suggested that, when making his lunch, he also make his wife's, reducing her stress at lunchtime. She agreed to concentrate on getting the evening meal organised. This meant doing the shopping and pre-preparing a meal or two on the weekend. Together they've found a way to play to their strengths, and found a solution.

It's important to identify what barriers might prevent you from having a more nutritious diet. For example, if you want to increase the quantity of vegetables you eat (an issue for most Australians) and you know lunchtime is where you fall down, what can you eat at lunch to boost your intake? You love a salad sandwich at lunchtime, but you never have this due to the preparation required, so usually opt for a ham and cheese toastie instead. What are the barriers to being prepared to make the salad sandwich? Is it that the ingredients are not in the fridge at home because you don't buy them when out shopping?

Here are some strategies to overcome the barriers in this example:

- » Put the necessary salad ingredients on the shopping list.
- » Prepare the salad in a container the night before, while making the evening meal.
- » Make a big bowl of salad at once, enough for a few days.
- » Buy the salad already prepared.
- » Take the salad ingredients to work at the start of the week and keep them in the fridge to use each day.
- » Swap the ham most days for another, less processed, source of protein, such as egg, canned fish, tofu, lean chicken, cheese, mashed beans, or other meat leftover from the night before.
- » Keep in the cheese for protein, calcium and taste. There's nothing better than melted cheese!

MAKING A PLAN

In summary, here are the steps I recommend you follow in order to take action:

- **Goals**: Write down what you would like to achieve (S.M.A.R.T goals). Make these specific to yourself. For example:
  - Improved energy levels after training and in games
  - Fuel myself so I can complete a certain sporting event or achieve a personal best (PB)
  - Reduce blood pressure (or another health marker)
  - Stop yo-yo dieting
  - Prepare more of my own food (based on knowing ingredients, quality, general health prevention)
- **Strategies**: What will you do to achieve these goals?
  - Planning – what and when do I need to plan in order to successfully do this?
  - Support – who will help me, for example to shop and cook?
- **Measure**: Monitor progress
  - Keep a diary for a few months describing how I feel – energy, stress levels
  - Visit the GP for a health check-up
  - Monitor spending to ensure more money is being spent on fresh produce and less on highly processed foods
  - Keep track of the number of home-cooked versus takeaway meals
  - Look at athletic performance – times, strength, achievements
  - Energy levels – getting up ready to start the day, feeling lethargic/energetic during the day or at training.

HELPING NEW AFL PLAYERS MAKE CHANGES

Each year we have a new group of first-year players join the AFL. They are generally around 18 years old, some living away from home for the first time, suddenly faced with having to make most of their food choices for themselves. Others live with a host family for a year or two, and have access to the food the family eats.

The players who have had nutrition education and have cooked at home have an advantage. There is so much to learn when you arrive at an AFL club, so if you already have your basic nutrition covered (and know its importance), that's one less thing to worry about. You know how to fuel yourself for the gruelling pre-season training.

For some, however, thinking about what they eat is a new concept. My job is to help them realise how important nutrition is for their performance as a professional athlete, and to develop their skills to achieve this. They will have body composition goals to meet, with skinfold tests tracking body fat levels, but also need to be fuelled to complete physical tasks.

To improve their knowledge and skills, I conduct practical sessions where I take them to the supermarket and show them what is available. We identify which foods are suitable for them and quick and easy to prepare. After a heavy training day they will be tired and hungry when they come home. Chopping up an array of vegetables for a stir-fry is unlikely to happen, so using the frozen variety can be a good solution.

I teach them how to read food labels, so they can make appropriate choices about breakfast cereals, canned foods, sauces, yoghurts, etc. Education helps facilitate long-term change.

We also hold cooking sessions in the kitchen at the club, and the boys cook. They are very competitive, and always want me to choose the best dish! Although I sometimes worry about them finishing with all their fingers intact, their confidence improves with the practice, making them more likely to prepare food at home.

A few years back I was teaching a player from the country who had minimal cooking skills. During the first cooking session he was getting frustrated about chopping carrots into strips for a stir-fry. He was not enjoying it at all! A year later, with some more sessions under his belt and plenty of practice at home, he told me he made homemade gnocchi (from scratch) for his parents when they came to visit. Amazing! Those skills will help him keep his nutrition on track way beyond his football career.

DEVELOPING COOKING SKILLS

Developing our cooking skills increases the likelihood that we will cook. Start your children cooking from a young age. Get them in the kitchen cooking, helping and also shopping. That way when they are living independently they won't be living on instant noodles and takeaway. It's much easier to carry on the good habits you have grown up with than to establish new ones. They may fall in love with cooking, and having their help will lighten your load. Cooking is like any skill: once you develop confidence in it, it transforms from an overwhelming task or chore to what can be a fun and rewarding pastime.

My daughter loves to cook desserts. Her creations are usually pieces of art: a beautifully decorated birthday cake, or, lately, savoury muffins for her school lunch. She is developing skills – reading the recipe, chopping, measuring, stirring, using the oven and the stove – and confidence in the kitchen. We talk about fuelling for her sport. It is a great way to develop a positive relationship with food. She has moved on to homemade ravioli and dumplings that we make together.

When my son was seventeen he stayed at a friend's house for a few nights with some mates. The parents were overseas, and though I was not fond of the idea at first, after setting some rules I agreed to it. I'm glad I did, as the thing he was most excited about was planning the menu for the evening meals! He asked me about dishes and the things he would need, and then they all went shopping together. The basic cooking he had done at home gave him the confidence to tackle this, and he loved it. He proudly whipped up homemade hamburgers, a chicken curry and pasta bolognaise (although he was less happy about doing the dishes). He's recently mastered beef bourguignon. At least I know he won't be living on takeaway when he moves out. My mother-in-law told me her advice to her son was that if you can read, you can cook. It's so true – get out a recipe and have a go!

CHAPTER 16

Making Life Easier in the Kitchen

People are often strapped for time, especially if they're trying to fit in training on top of work and general life. Preparing healthy food to meet performance goals is critical, but it takes time, so let's look at ways we can make life a little easier. There are plenty of foods you can include that are nutritious and save some preparation time.

CANNED FOODS

Many people think canned foods have no nutritional value. Wrong! Canned food is an important part of our food supply, making it possible to have a wide range of fruits and vegetables all year round, and at a reasonable price. They can be conveniently stored in cupboards at home or on your desk at work, making it easier to increase the amount of fruit and vegetables we eat.

PRESERVATIVES?

Contrary to what people often think, canned foods generally have very little if any preservatives added. The can acts like a small pressure cooker, sealed and airtight. Once opened, canned foods should be treated as if fresh, and used within a few days. Many canned vegetables have salt added, which does act as a preservative, but you can rinse it away.

IS CANNED FOOD SAFE TO EAT?

Don't store any remaining food in the can once it's been opened – the acidity of the opened canned food can cause some of the minerals from the can to transfer into the food. Always decant the food into a glass or plastic container and refrigerate it.

Many people worry that canned foods pose a health risk due to bisphenol A (BPA). BPA is a chemical found in the lining of cans (and in some plastic food containers) that is used to extend the shelf life of food, and to protect it from contamination. A small amount of BPA may leach out of the lining and into the food. The levels of BPA we can be exposed to from eating canned food are deemed safe by Food Standards Australia New Zealand. You would have to eat large amounts of canned food every day to reach an amount that would be toxic.

CANNED FISH

Canned fish has grown in popularity over recent years. Quick, convenient, and an economical source of protein, vitamin D and omega 3 fats, it's perfect for lunches, evening meals or a snack. No refrigeration is required, unlike with many other protein-containing foods, so you can take cans of fish to eat pre- or post-training, when travelling to competitions or as extras in a school lunch. Read the labels to check the omega 3 fatty acid levels as these vary between brands. Choose those with the highest levels of omega 3, as these healthy fats are essential, can't be made by the body and can help reduce inflammation, as well as providing other heart health benefits. Sardines and mackerel are rich in beneficial omega 3 fatty acids – try some of the new flavoured varieties.

Vary the types of canned fish you eat, as fish can contain small amounts of heavy metals, particularly mercury. Food Standards Australia New Zealand recommend one 95-gram can of tuna per day as being safe to eat, assuming no other fish is eaten. If you also eat fresh fish, you may like to skip the can of tuna or other canned fish that day.

During pregnancy, it's safe to eat 2–3 serves of most fish types per week, including canned tuna or salmon. Pregnant women should limit fish with high levels of mercury, including shark (flake), marlin, swordfish and orange roughy/deep sea perch.

SODIUM AND SUGAR LEVELS IN CANNED FOOD

Read the labels so you're aware of the salt (sodium) content in the canned item, as well as any sugar that may have been added. There are many low- or reduced-salt options available, and rinsing the contents can reduce the salt content by half. Choosing canned fish in oil rather than brine can also reduce sodium levels – read nutrition panels on labels (see page 194). If eating canned food after being active, the sodium can help replace sodium that has been lost through sweat, so it's not all bad – some of us need the sodium.

Some canned foods, such as baked beans, contain a small amount of added sugar, but the benefit of the nutrients in the beans outweighs this. Canned legumes (peas, beans, lentils) can be a great addition to a meal, particularly for a vegetarian athlete, providing protein, fibre, carbohydrate, vitamins and minerals. For example, you can add legumes to salad, soup, casserole or chilli con carne, mash them, make a dip (e.g. hummus) or eat them straight from the can. They are quick, nutritious, portable, economical, and don't require refrigeration. Look out for new varieties, including black beans, which are delicious in a bolognaise pasta sauce, or pinto beans for Mexican dishes.

The starch you can see in the liquid in canned legumes can pass undigested to the large intestine and be fermented into gas, causing bloating and discomfort in some people. Rinsing the legumes helps remove some of this starch. For those who don't mind it, you can also use this liquid to thicken a casserole or stew.

Fruit is generally peeled before canning, so you miss out on the fibre from the peel, and, yes, it does contain sugar, but the fruit is still packed with nutrients. Make a quick nutritious dessert using canned fruit in juice rather than syrup, or tip out the juice and top with yoghurt. Canned fruit is convenient to keep in the cupboard, and can be handy for lots of things, such as:

- » when you're travelling and fresh fruit might not be readily available
- » to add to smoothies, particularly if you need to increase energy intake
- » an easy-to-digest, pre-, post- or mid-competition carbohydrate snack
- » an easy-to-chew snack for when you're tired after training or during a long event, e.g. during a long day of cycling, a long walk or a hike.

I have found the snack packs of fruit particularly appealing to swimmers who need to fuel themselves between events over a long day – this is a time when the higher sugar content is appropriate. The same could apply for competitors at the athletics track. A container can also easily be added to muesli and yoghurt for an energy-packed breakfast – perfect for travelling athletes staying in hotel rooms with minimal meal preparation equipment.

Using some canned foods in your diet can help add variety and convenience without compromising on nutrition. I choose Australian-grown products where possible, as I have confidence in the farming practices.

TIPS FOR INCLUDING CANNED FOODS IN YOUR DIET

- » Baked beans at breakfast
- » Kidney beans added to bolognaise sauce or chilli con carne
- » Chickpeas added to a casserole or curry
- » Any canned beans added to a salad – add some canned fish and corn for a meal
- » Corn kernels added to a salad, to a frittata, as a side vegetable, in a stir-fry or in soup (I like chicken and sweet corn)
- » Tomatoes added to pasta sauces, ratatouille, or cooked up with eggs and spinach for breakfast

- » Baby beets straight from the can for a sweet snack, on sandwiches, in salads, or with curries as a side vegetable
- » Fruit such as pears poached for dessert, on top of cereal with yoghurt for a snack, or in smoothies, pancakes and muffins
- » Sardines, tuna, salmon or mackerel added to sandwiches, eaten on their own, in salads, with rice and vegetables, in patties or with pasta

FROZEN FOODS

The frozen foods that make it into my trolley are mainly vegetables, some fruit, a litre or two of ice cream, and maybe a few dumplings and some filo pastry. Some of the frozen meals might be okay on occasion, but I wouldn't have them as a staple. If choosing a frozen meal, read the labels to ensure the product contains adequate protein, carbohydrate and vegetables for your needs. Watch for sodium, which can be very high – this is good if you need a boost, but not on an everyday basis. Frozen meals can be handy and nutritious at times, just be selective.

I make sure I always have some frozen vegetables in my freezer – peas, corn, beans, some mixed vegetables, and sometimes oven chips. Frozen vegetables are snap frozen, meaning they are picked and go straight to the packing and freezing facility with little time for nutrient loss. I only buy Australian-grown vegetables. Read the packets to find out where the product was grown (not where it was packed). 'Product of [country name inserted]' doesn't mean the vegetables were grown there – in some cases they may be imported products that were packed in that country, but not grown there. Australian horticulture standards are high, but that's not the case everywhere. This, along with wanting to support farmers and reduce food miles, is why I buy Australian.

> ## TIPS FOR USING FROZEN VEGETABLES
>
> » Have corn cobs for a carbohydrate boost before or after training.
> » Throw mixed frozen vegetables in chilli con carne, homemade fried rice, noodles, a shepherd's pie or soup.
> » Add peas. I love baby ones, as they are sweet and can even be added frozen to a salad with tuna, corn and rice, or have them as side vegetables with mashed potato.
> » When vegetables are out of season, using frozen varieties can give greater choice and be more economical. For example, I use green beans and cauliflower with cheese (for protein) to go with my roast.
> » Add mixed frozen vegetables to a meal to save time and fill you up.

BECOMING A SLICK SHOPPER

How many times have you found yourself wanting to cook something only to realise that you don't have all the ingredients? Or got home from training or work to find the fridge and cupboards bare? Rather than making do, some forward planning can have you eating what your body needs to optimally prepare for upcoming events.

Think of shopping as part of your training. Fuelling yourself is an important part of the overall picture. Schedule in time to shop, or liaise with other household members to make sure someone has it on their agenda.

It is human nature to throw items into the trolley or basket quickly when we start shopping and then slow down. To ensure this works in your favour, start with the outer part of the supermarket first, where the fresh produce is, and enter the aisles last.

MAKE GROCERY SHOPPING FUN

Grocery shopping can get monotonous, so here are some ways to spice it up:

- » Visit fresh food markets/weekend markets.
- » Make it social, meeting up with friends while shopping.
- » Walk to the shops, to turn it into exercise.
- » Take turns doing the shopping, so everyone in the household contributes.
- » Make it an outing by driving somewhere different to shop.
- » Shop together and allocate each person a few items on the list – see who gets their list done first.
- » Pick a time when you are likely to enjoy it, rather than feeling rushed.
- » Order your groceries online and have them delivered.
- » Pick one new dish each week to get you excited about getting different ingredients.

UNDERSTANDING FOOD LABELS – HOW DO I KNOW WHAT TO BUY?

There are so many different nutrition-related claims on the packaging of supermarket products that these can quickly become confusing. The nutrition panel gives you a breakdown of the nutrients in the product, but it's good to read the list of ingredients, too. Are they ingredients you know and want to eat? The ingredients will be listed from largest in quantity to smallest.

If you want the full run-down on the regulations regarding food labelling, visit the Food Standards Australia New Zealand Code website. It explains what claims can be used, and what level of nutrients a product must contain to be allowed to make that claim. It also explains what the numbers you see on packages relate to; for example, 955 means the sweetener sucralose. If you are limiting the amount of packaged food you eat you will not need to spend too much time on this. There is a good mobile app called Food Switch, which helps you determine whether a food is high in fat, salt, sugar, fibre and some other nutrients. You simply scan the barcode of the package and it gives a traffic light system report: red means beware, orange means caution and green means good. It also suggests alternative brands within that food range. The app was developed in Australia by the George Institute in Sydney.

Things to consider when reading labels on food packets include:

DIETARY FIBRE

In general, we want to eat foods that are high in dietary fibre. At some times, however, you may want low-fibre foods, such as when competing in sports that require you to weigh in before an event, or when you are on the border of making weight. When buying a breakfast cereal, a good guide is usually to find one that is a 'source of fibre' or high in dietary fibre (contains 8 grams or more per 100 grams). When looking for low fibre, you may choose a cereal containing less than 5 grams per 100 grams.

SODIUM

For general health, aim for foods that contain less than 300 milligrams of sodium per 100 grams.

Food Standards Australia New Zealand Code classifies food as being:

» low salt when it contains less than 120 milligrams per 100 grams
» high salt when it contains 400 milligrams or more per 100 grams.

Remember that people who are training and losing a considerable amount of sodium in sweat may not require these constraints. Sodium intake is very individual, and sodium guidelines are based on the average person's requirements, not an athlete's.

FAT

You can determine where fat is coming from by reading the ingredients list. Avoid foods with hydrogenated oils, palm oil, and foods that list '**vegetable oil**', as this is likely to be palm or a blend of lower-quality oils. If manufacturers are using a good-quality oil such as extra virgin olive oil, they will want to tell you, and will state this on the label.

The claim '**baked not fried**' is often misinterpreted as meaning the product is low in fat. Foods that have been 'baked not fried' can still contain plenty of fat, and, more importantly, this claim fails to mention the type of fat used. Was the food baked in poor-quality oil, listed as 'vegetable oil', or a good-quality extra virgin olive oil? Poor-quality oils are more likely to contribute to inflammation, while good-quality extra virgin olive oils may help reduce this.

'**Low in fat**' means the product can't contain more than a certain level of fat for that particular food category, as stated in the Food Standards Australia New Zealand Code. The level changes for different foods. Low-fat cheese, for example, often contains 10 per cent fat, while low-fat milk contains 2 per cent or less. It depends on what the standard fat level for that food usually is.

'**Reduced fat**' means the food contains a certain percentage less than the standard level of fat. A reduced-fat tasty cheese, for example, usually contains 25 per cent less fat than full-fat cheese, which is around 35 per cent fat. That means the reduced-fat version contains around 10 per cent less fat, which is still 25 per cent fat. In this case, I would buy the standard cheese and enjoy the taste and overall nutritional value it provides. The quality of fat and the overall nutritional value of the food are more important than the total fat content alone.

SUGAR

Sugar can be added in many forms, so it's important to read both the ingredient listing and the nutrition panel. If there seems to be more sugar in a product than you might have expected, make sure you can identify where it has come from. Fruit or dairy will contribute to the sugar percentage, but also provide beneficial nutrients, unlike sugar that has been added on its own. Sugars can take many different forms, such as glucose syrups, fructose concentrates, fruit juice concentrates, rice syrups, dextrose ... Anything ending in 'ose' refers to a sugar of some type in its chemical name.

The claim **'no added sugar'**, often seen on fruit juices or yoghurts, can be confusing. It means no sucrose (table sugar) has been added. It does not mean that the product is low in sugar or free of sugar. For example, some yoghurts are sweetened with fruit juice concentrates, which is essentially the same as adding sugar. Fruit naturally contains sugar, so fruit juice concentrate is very high in sugar. Check the ingredients list to see if fruit juice concentrate has been included. Nutritionally, this is the same as adding sucrose (table sugar). For people who have a fructose intolerance (fruit juice is higher in fructose than sucrose is), this can also contribute to bloating and gut issues.

It is difficult to say what level of sugar is acceptable in a packaged food, because it's not just the total sugar that matters, it's where the sugar comes from. Is it from added fruit, such as dried fruit in cereal, which brings other valuable nutrients with it? In general, look for products containing less than 10 per cent sugar (10 grams in 100 grams), or less than ~20 per cent if the food contains a significant amount of fruit. For flavoured yoghurts, a good guide is less than 12 per cent sugar.

The sugar content of each product needs to be looked at individually. Consider:

- the food's overall nutritional value, not just sugar in isolation
- when the food is going to be eaten, i.e. fruit yoghurt eaten by a teenager before swimming training might be beneficial because it provides extra kilojoules, carbohydrate and protein, is tasty and is convenient to have in the fridge at home, no preparation required
- how often the food will be eaten, e.g. I give AFL footballers pikelets with jam, which are high in sugar and have minimal other nutritional value, on game day only. At other times, a food that provides more nutritional value and is lower in sugar would be chosen for a snack.

CHOLESTEROL FREE

One day I was in the supermarket and saw an elderly couple shopping together. The gentleman placed some honey in the trolley and his wife quickly took it out, telling him he couldn't have the honey because it didn't say 'cholesterol free' on the label. It would be inappropriate for honey to make that claim, because honey is pure sugar – it doesn't have anything to do with fat or cholesterol. All honey is cholesterol free.

'Cholesterol free' is an irrelevant claim because the amount of cholesterol in foods is small. What affects your cholesterol level is the amount and type of fat in the product, which your liver might use to produce cholesterol. Avoiding trans, hydrogenated and in most cases saturated fats (particularly if from palm oil and processed foods), and choosing foods containing predominately monounsaturated, fats is more important. Look at the overall nutritional value of the food, and don't worry about the 'cholesterol free' claim.

GLUTEN FREE

Gluten-free foods have become very popular, but many people don't really understand what it means. Gluten free simply means the product contains no gluten. Marketers have been putting this claim all over products, as people seem to think gluten-free food is a healthier option – in fact, it is often the opposite. Avoiding gluten is only important for those with gluten or sometimes wheat intolerances. Gluten is a protein in wheat and some other cereals that is perfectly suitable to eat, provided you don't have an intolerance. Don't get sucked into marketing claims that may not be relevant to you (and that increase the price of a product significantly).

MUESLI BARS

Muesli bars are a good example of the importance of reading the label when making your choice. They're a great snack for travelling, or before or after sport, but in general you'd be better off grabbing a rolled oat-based breakfast cereal with milk, or a handful of trail mix (nuts, seeds, dried fruit). Most muesli bars are stuck together with sugars. Yoghurt-topped muesli bars have a particularly high sugar content – the 'yoghurt' on top is usually a mix of vegetable oil and sugar, which I would consider to be an icing. Leave those ones on the shelf.

That said, muesli bars can be a good option on competition day. Before or after a game they're a great supply of carbohydrate, with some slow-release carbohydrate from the oats and quick-release carbohydrate from the glucose, honey and other added sugars you might find. I look for muesli bars with minimal ingredients. More ingredients often equals more sugar added, and it's best to have most ingredients from whole grains (e.g. oats, triticale, quinoa) and/or nuts.

Muesli bars tend to be high in kilojoules, often containing around 750 kilojoules per bar, which is equivalent to two slices of bread. One muesli bar rarely fills a hungry person; there are more filling and nutritious choices available.

Some muesli bars claim to be 'high protein'. This can be from added protein powder, rather than from food ingredients such as nuts or seeds (as you may expect). If a muesli bar contains added protein powder I won't use them with elite athletes, because I can't easily check where the protein powder has been sourced from, or whether it has been tested to ensure it is free from World Anti-Doping Authority (WADA)–banned substances. Even for athletes who are not being drug tested, I still prefer protein from wholefood ingredients such as nuts, legumes, or seeds. Check the labels and make sure you know what you're eating.

SHOPPING LISTS

I always recommend making a shopping list. There are many benefits:

- » A shopping list helps keep you on track, saving time and money.
- » You can have a standard list that you add to each week, and change according to the season, to be efficient.
- » A list can help increase your vegetable intake: start the list with the vegetables rather than the meats or protein alternatives.
- » Think about the meals you will make as you write the list, to ensure you buy ingredients that will work together. Consider which days you may need more carbohydrate for recovery or before games or events and what meals you like then (you may have favourites). Remember to cater for lunch and breakfast too.
- » Having a shopping list means you are less likely to run out of foods like milk or cereal, meaning you can always eat a healthy breakfast and pre-prepare your lunch.
- » To save time, group foods based on the shops or markets.

Shopping for food can be enjoyable! After all, you are picking the foods that are going to fuel your body and tantalise your tastebuds.

STAPLES FOR THE FRIDGE, FREEZER AND PANTRY

- » Greenery – fresh salad mix, spinach leaves, silverbeet, lettuce or rocket
- » A selection of in-season vegetables (choose a variety of colours, as this will ensure a range of nutrients)

- Frozen vegetables – corn, spinach, peas, beans
- Frozen berries or other fruit
- Fresh, in-season fruit – two pieces per person per day
- Wholegrain bread – for variety have wraps, English muffins, rolls, etc.
- Wholegrain breakfast cereals – oats, muesli, wheat biscuits, quinoa flakes (gluten free, if needed)
- Wholegrain dry biscuits
- Spreads – yeast extract spread (Vegemite), 100 per cent peanut butter or other nut spread
- Eggs
- Yoghurt (mostly natural)
- Milk
- Cheese – tasty, ricotta, cottage, feta
- Canned fish – tuna, sardines, salmon
- Canned vegetables and fruit – corn, legumes, beetroot, tomatoes, kidney beans, chickpeas, baked beans, pineapple, pears
- Pasta, couscous (wholemeal varieties are available)
- Rice (preferably brown), rice noodles
- Other grains and legumes, such as quinoa, freekeh, barley, dried soup mix, lentils
- Condiments – balsamic vinegar, extra virgin olive oil, soy sauce, mustard, herbs, spices, curry pastes
- Meat and seafood

This list is by no means exhaustive. You can add and subtract your favourites and change it with the seasons. I also like to have a fruit toast in the freezer for when I want a sweet treat, and a little stash of dark chocolate.

CHAPTER 17
Quick Meal Ideas

BREAKFAST

Breakfast is my favourite meal of the day! I am always hungry in the morning, and eating breakfast gets me set for the day. Over the years, the traditional breakfast routine has changed. Instead of sitting together at the table, these days many people are grabbing a coffee on the run and eating at work or at varying times during the morning. (Breakfast doesn't have to be first thing in the morning if you don't feel hungry then – choose a time that suits you.) It has also become popular to eat breakfast out on weekends, holidays and after a fun run or bike ride. Give a little thought to what you choose for breakfast to start your day.

Breakfasts can vary from nutrient poor to nutrient rich. For instance, a breakfast of white bread, butter and jam is low in dietary fibre, protein, vitamins and minerals, and high in quickly digested carbohydrates (high GI). This might be a suitable breakfast when you need quickly released carbohydrate before a race, but not for a healthy standard breakfast. Wholegrain toast topped with cheese, avocado and tomato is higher in dietary fibre, protein, vitamins and minerals and provides slow-release carbohydrate. Try to make your breakfast a nutritionally packed meal. For those who don't feel like having an early breakfast, plan a nutritious mid-morning snack, as you are likely to be ravenous by then. It's all about planning.

NUTRITIONAL BENEFITS OF BREAKFAST

A good breakfast offers loads of nutritional benefits:

- » It breaks the fast from the night before, which is particularly important for those wishing to gain muscle mass.
- » It may be a recovery meal after morning exercise.
- » It can be fuel before morning exercise.
- » It can give a good fibre boost, e.g. wholegrain cereals, wholegrain breads, fruit, vegetables.
- » It assists in meeting calcium requirements, e.g. milk, fortified beverages, yoghurt.
- » It boosts your concentration, particularly for children (it's hard to concentrate if you're hungry).

On the other hand, skipping breakfast means it is a long time between protein intake from dinner the night before and protein foods at lunchtime.

BREAKFAST IDEAS FOR HOME OR THE CAFE

- **Cereals**
  - natural muesli
  - porridge – rolled oats or barley and oats
  - cereals – choose a variety that contains more than 7 grams of dietary fibre per 100 grams, and have it with cow's milk, fermented milk drinks or added-calcium soy
  - Bircher muesli (made with natural yoghurt; you can make a week's worth in advance)
  - add fresh fruit or frozen fruit (e.g. mango, berries), dried fruit (in small quantities), or canned fruit (drain the juice away)

- **Yoghurt**
  - Natural yoghurt is generally best – add your own fruit, nuts, seeds and oats for flavour. Some flavoured yoghurts can be low in sugar (10 per cent or less per 100 grams). Protein and calcium levels vary greatly, so read labels, particularly if you're using breakfast as a recovery meal and want to hit the 20+ grams of protein mark in the meal.

- **Bread/toast**

  Try heavy wholegrain or sourdough rye breads, toasting muffins, wholegrain fruit loaf or wholemeal crumpets topped with:
  - avocado, cheese and Vegemite
  - ricotta or feta cheese with tomato, sprinkled with black pepper and fresh basil
  - 100 per cent nut spreads
  - ricotta cheese, banana, crushed nuts and a drizzle of honey. Add a glass of milk or have a latte for protein.
  - sardines, tomato and lemon juice
  - cut up fresh or dried fruit and eat it with nuts or cheese, and some wholegrain crackers. This can be prepared the night before.

- **Cooked breakfast**

  A cooked breakfast can be more than eggs on toast, and can be quick and easy, too. Remember to add vegetables. Ideas include:
  - Spinach, asparagus, mushrooms, grilled tomatoes, corn, roasted or grilled capsicums, baked beans, cannellini beans, rocket or kale.
  - Heat up a bowl or mug of soup.
  - Hard-boiled eggs, baby cucumbers and cherry tomatoes. Pre-boil a few eggs in advance and store them in the fridge.
  - Pancakes – try including ricotta cheese or quark yoghurt and wholemeal flour in the batter, and have yoghurt and fruit for topping. Make extra batter for the next day.
  - Savoury pancakes are a great option too.
  - Corn and spinach or zucchini fritters, with grilled tomato and smoked salmon. The fritters taste great when cold with salad or in a sandwich. They are perfect for a pre- or post-training snack at any time of the day.
  - Bacon – good protein. It's fine to have the occasional rasher of bacon or ham, but note that these are salty processed meats, so only have them every now and again.

- **Spreads and toppings**

  There are plenty of alternatives to butter and margarine that offer more nutrients. More nutrient-rich choices include:
  - Avocado, tomato, ricotta, feta, bocconcini or tasty cheese, nut spreads, drizzle of extra virgin olive oil, pesto.
  - Smoked salmon – it boasts omega 3 fats, as do sardines and tuna. Smoked salmon doesn't need any preparation, you can eat it straight from the packet as a protein boost.

RUN OUT OF TIME TO MAKE BREAKFAST?

If you find yourself skipping breakfast because you're short on time, try these strategies:

» Set the alarm clock 10 minutes earlier.
» Set out the cereal pack and bowl (or whatever you plan to eat) the night before.
» Have a bowl of fruit and tub of yoghurt ready in the fridge.
» Keep pre-made hard-boiled eggs in the fridge and have them with a glass of milk.
» Eat a can of beans straight from the can.
» Take breakfast ingredients to work, or keep them there so you can eat when you arrive.
» Delegate to someone who has more time in the morning to prepare your breakfast (you can do something in return for them at another time).

LUNCH IDEAS

Being prepared can make it easier to bring nutritious lunches from home, which can also be lighter on the wallet. There are numerous choices for lunch. Some will fuel you for the rest of the day, while others can make you feel sluggish and want to nap. Here are a few ideas:

» **Salad:** Try a salad that includes more than just greens; add protein to keep you full, such as eggs or a can of beans or fish. If time is a constraint you can buy partly prepared salads at the supermarket, such as a salad bowl or pre-sliced vegetables.

- **Soup:** One of my favourite lunches is a good, hearty soup. Soup is such a great way to increase your vegetable intake and stay hydrated. Include protein to help spread your protein intake out over the day.

    Choose the amount of carbohydrate to suit your energy expenditure and add accordingly: potato, pasta, rice, noodles, or a crusty bread roll. Soup can be a saviour for athletes with body weight restrictions, as you can choose a vegetable base that is filling and then add protein and carbohydrate (noodles, rice) based on your needs. Homemade or even supermarket-bought soup can be a handy afternoon snack or evening meal, too. Make soup in big batches and freeze. Some good options include:

    - minestrone (beans, pasta, vegetables)
    - beef and barley (or other carbohydrate)
    - chicken and sweet corn
    - lentil.

- **Homemade pizza:** When eating pizza, it can be easy to eat too much carbohydrate, due to the base, and not enough protein and vegetables. A side dish of salad, an entree of soup and vegetables, and toppings of tomato, spinach, capsicum, mushrooms, eggplant and rocket can all help boost the vegetables. Toppings such as chicken, prawns, smoked salmon, lamb and cheese will add some protein, and a thin wrap can make for an easy base. Think of the pizza toppings as a variation on a sandwich.

- **Leftovers:** Cooking extra food the night before and taking it to work saves preparation time. Try to keep a balance of carbohydrate, protein and vegetables, though, rather than just having what is left over.

- **Sandwiches:** It's hard to beat a good sandwich for convenience, price (if making your own), nutrition and taste. Think about the three components needed: carbohydrate, protein and, most importantly, vegetables. Have these available to add to your sandwich and stack the vegetable filling so it's as thick (or thicker) than the two slices of bread. To make this quick, prepare a container of salad vegetables with enough for a few days of sandwich making. It saves pulling everything out of the fridge each time.

TIPS FOR A NOURISHING SANDWICH OR WHOLEGRAIN WRAP

- **Salad:** At least three salad items
  - e.g. beetroot, lettuce, tomato, baby spinach, rocket, mushroom, bean shoots, carrot, cucumber, onion, avocado, roasted pumpkin, capsicum, sundried tomatoes, eggplant
- **Protein:** At least one protein source
  - e.g. chicken (no skin), turkey, lean beef, fish (salmon, tuna, sardines), egg, legumes (e.g. smashed beans), marinated tofu, cottage cheese, tasty cheese
- **Condiments:** Add flavour to your sandwich with fresh herbs and flavourings
  - e.g. mustard, pickles, hummus, olive tapenade, cracked black pepper, coriander, basil, chilli, oregano
- **Bread:** Vary the breads so you don't get bored
  - choose wholegrain or heavy dark rye, spelt bread and sourdough (spelt and sourdough can be easier to digest for some people). Eating a large bread roll is like eating three slices of bread, so adjust according to your needs.

Toasting your sandwich is appealing in winter – just remember to also add a vegetable filling to your 'toastie'. It should contain more than just ham and cheese!

If you have a sweet tooth, you might like to finish lunch with fruit salad and a spoonful of yoghurt, or save it for the afternoon.

If you get hungry at around 11 am, have an early lunch instead of snacking. You can then have a second lunch (or the other half of your early lunch) mid-afternoon rather than more snack foods, which can be low in nutritional value.

THE EVENING MEAL

'What's for dinner?' That must be one of the most common questions we ask ourselves or those who prepare it for us. I asked my mum this question every day when I was young, and my daughter still asks me now. Deciding what to prepare each night can be a chore. Making a nutritious evening meal doesn't mean it needs to be restaurant standard or take hours to prepare.

Cooking at home is worthwhile; research shows that when people eat at home, they have smaller portion sizes with more vegetables and less salt. Think of it as more than just a meal – it's a time to catch up with others in the household, or to invite friends over for a catch-up. It is also an opportunity to model healthy eating behaviours, try new foods and choose nutritious meals. When you cook your own food, you know what is in the food, such as:

- » quality and type of oil – choose fresh extra virgin olive oil over lower-quality oils
- » lean cuts of meat, fresh seafood
- » more vegetables
- » wholegrain breads
- » less added sugar and salt.

And as an added bonus, cooking at home is better for the budget, too.

PLANNING THE EVENING MEAL

Plan your meal with vegetables in mind, not just the protein source. Including vegetables or salad at each meal is a great habit to get into. Then think about the protein and carbohydrate you'll add to the vegetables. As a guide, aim to fill between one-third and half of your plate with vegetables, and one-quarter to one-third with protein and carbohydrate, depending on your individual needs. An active person is likely to need more protein and carbohydrate, so should have one-third of each option, while a more sedentary person should have half a plate of vegetables. Some nights you might need more protein, others more carbohydrate or vegetable.

- » Have a plan for the week so you can shop for the ingredients needed all at once.
- » Develop specialty dishes, with each household member becoming familiar with a few meals they can prepare confidently and quickly on their night to cook.
- » Choose a night to try new dishes – maybe every second weekend. When a new dish has been mastered it could be added to the general repertoire.

SUITING THE WHOLE FAMILY

The last thing you want to be doing is cooking numerous meals to meet everyone's desires. I often help clients work out how to avoid this. Here are some tips to try:

- » Make the food visually inviting – kids particularly love bright colours.
  - » Try stir-fries with brightly coloured vegetables such as carrots, capsicum, snow peas, corn, asparagus.
  - » Have a fresh fruit platter on the table for after dinner.
- » Engage the household in planning and preparing meals.
  - » Having input into the upcoming menu results in greater acceptance. When people help prepare the food, it gives them ownership of it.
- » Some of us prefer vegetables raw rather than cooked.
  - » snow peas, mushrooms, celery and frozen peas can all be delicious raw.
- » Include a maximum of one or two new foods in a meal.
  - » Introduce new flavours gradually.

- » One rejection doesn't mean they don't like the meal – it might take a few tries to get used to the smell, look, taste and texture. Science shows that it can take ten or more tries to like a new food.
- » Alternate between people's favourite dishes so everyone gets a go.

Cooking takes confidence and the willingness to have a go. The more confident you feel, the more likely you'll be to cook, meaning you'll have less takeaway and be more willing to try new foods.

 ## TIME-SAVERS

A common issue my clients encounter is getting home from work or training late and feeling exhausted, and needing to have a healthy meal ready quickly. To overcome this challenge, develop a plan with strategies that will work for you.

- » Ask for help with meal preparation to make it quicker and easier.
- » Cook extra on weekends and freeze or refrigerate for later in the week.
- » Chop more vegetables one night to cook fresh in a different dish the next night, e.g. stir-fry one night, curry the next.
- » Add different herbs and spices to give an easy-to-prepare dish a different flavour.
- » Use a mix of fresh and frozen vegetables to save preparation and shopping time and to add variety.
- » Buy the meat already cut into strips, if time is of the essence.
- » Set the slow cooker in the morning, or overnight, ready for the evening meal.

- » Wake up early to cut vegetables or prepare a salad and put it in the fridge.
- » Marinate meat, fish or tofu the night before, or in the morning.
- » Cook pasta sauce the night before, after you have already eaten and had some time to recharge. You might get a second wind to cook the next night's dinner. If you have a later start, cook before going to work.
- » Some foods, such as curries, are often tastier the day after, so they're great to make in advance.
- » Easy-to-prepare home-cooked meals are quicker, cheaper and more nutritious than most takeaway options. For example:
  - » Make an omelette.
  - » Warm up soup.
  - » Make a sandwich/toasted sandwich or hamburger with plenty of salad, using wholegrain bread.
  - » Boil the kettle to make couscous, then add a can of tuna, corn and fresh spinach.
  - » Oven bake frozen chips, grill or barbecue a piece of fish, and open a bag of prepared mixed salad such as Asian slaw.

You will feel a whole lot better for it!

QUICK MEAL IDEAS

The following meal ideas are based around vegetables, one carbohydrate and a protein source. Quantities can then be adjusted for individual needs, which can change from day to day. Try these ideas to boost your menu:

- » baked fish (wrap in foil and everyone can add their own flavours, e.g. lemon, chilli, ginger, garlic, soy sauce), roasted potatoes (cut in quarters and brushed with extra virgin olive oil), three vegetables
- » lean grilled steak, or omelette, corn on the cob, sweet potato and greens
- » stir-fried chicken with brown rice and three or more vegetables
- » chicken (or chickpea) and vegetable curry (you can use a jar paste) with couscous, quinoa or brown rice
- » lean beef or legume bolognaise – spinach and pine nuts can be a nice addition for a change
- » chilli con carne or burritos (kangaroo mince makes a delicious sauce), with salad and rice
- » falafels or marinated beef or lamb kebabs with souvlaki bread and salad
- » seafood marinara or risotto – add spinach or a rocket side salad
- » marinated prawns on a mixed green salad with feta cheese
- » roast meat and roast vegetables – potato, mushrooms, pumpkin, capsicum, carrots, parsnip and onion
- » kangaroo burgers or vegetable burgers (e.g. lentil) piled with salad.

HEALTHY BARBECUE IDEAS

Barbecuing is a handy cooking method and a great extension of the usual kitchen. Cooking on the barbecue often becomes a social occasion, too. What comes to mind when you think about food on a barbecue? Sausages, steak, hamburgers. Everything meat focused. How about we add colour and nutrients by adding vegetables? Try capsicum, corn, mushrooms, zucchini, tomatoes, asparagus, potatoes, sweet potato, pumpkin – they're all great for the barbecue.

Serve up half of your plate with vegetables first, then add your meat, seafood, eggs or lentil burger. Barbecued food can make a quick meal to be enjoyed any time of the year. Not only is it healthier to have more vegetables on your barbecue, it's more economical too, especially if you choose vegetables that are in season.

Salads are a great accompaniment for a barbecue. Experiment with various vegetables: broccoli, cauliflower, snow pea sprouts, watercress and other leafy greens. You could add a whole grain or legume as a base, such as rice, quinoa, couscous, freekeh or chickpeas, to complete the meal.

Game meats such as kangaroo do well on the barbecue and are very lean, contain omega 3 fats and are a rich source of iron and zinc, too. I have tried crocodile, camel burgers and camel sausages, which are all quite delicious. Vary what you have, and try something new.

I suggest using extra virgin olive oil and adding herbs, both for flavour and the nutrients they provide. Try rosemary on potatoes, oregano, basil or coriander in salads and cracked black pepper and garlic on just about anything.

It can be tempting to eat straight off the barbecue, but this makes it very easy to overeat. It is best to serve up, sit down and enjoy.

Avoid charring the food, as this can increase the level of carcinogens in the meat and vegetables. Eating one burnt sausage won't cause a health issue, but regularly eating charred food is not recommended.

A barbecue is a great way to get more people involved with cooking. My teenage son, Matthew, likes to cook, so on Melbourne Cup day a few years back when we were having friends over, I gave him the utensils, meat and vegetables, a little guidance and asked him to cook the food on the barbecue. After a little hesitation, he took on the challenge and cooked a fantastic meal of meat and heaps of vegetables. These days he's a whizz in the kitchen.

TIPS FOR MAKING A HEALTHIER MEAL

- Remove fat from meat and skin from chicken before cooking.
- Cook seafood at least once a week, e.g. stir-fry prawns, barbecue fish or cook it in the oven, add salmon, sardines or tuna to pasta, add fish to stir-fries, curries or patties.
- Have at least three types of vegetables/salad items (not including potatoes).
- Add legumes (e.g. chickpeas, kidney beans, lentils) to soups and casseroles for protein, carbohydrate and fibre.
- Consider a meat-free dish once a week or more, using plant sources of protein instead.
- Use extra virgin olive oil as your main oil.
- Use vinegar in dressings.
- Use evaporated milk or yoghurt instead of cream for more calcium and protein.
- Freeze soup for dinners, snacks, or lunches.
- Frozen vegetables are still healthy and can save time.
- Add fresh herbs to dishes to increase flavour and nutrients (they are very high in antioxidants) and freeze extras in snap lock bags or containers (they will discolour, but that doesn't matter).

CHAPTER 18
How to Successfully Eat Out

Eating out is a great social activity that we all want to be able to enjoy. It is usually about more than the food you are eating – it's about the occasion. Many teams I have worked with (both sporting and corporate) have regular team lunches and dinners. It promotes team bonding, just like eating out with your friends. 'Breaking bread together' refers to more than just eating; it's about sharing a common bond and creating meaningful connection and cooperation.

How often you eat out will determine the importance of choosing wisely from the menu. If you only do this once every few weeks you can choose what you like, but if it's more than once a week you'll need to be more selective. With some thought, knowledge and planning, eating out regularly (which some of us do due to travel, our jobs, for team and family bonding, or because we simply enjoy it) can still work for you.

Have nights where you simply choose what you feel like and others where you base your choice on what will help with performance goals and health.

WHICH MENU ITEMS ARE SUITED TO ME?

In preparation for eating out it can pay to do a little homework. Check out the menu online before you go, or ring and ask some questions so you can make your choice in advance. Prior contact also gives the restaurant an opportunity to think about how they can accommodate you, which avoids the stress of being put on the spot when ordering. Don't be scared to ask for modifications to menu items. You are the customer – ask for what suits you.

Some things you could request to make a menu item more suitable could include:

- » Extra vegetables or salad to help fill you up and balance the meal.
- » Swapping chips for jacket or mashed potatoes. Or, if you feel like chips, what about requesting just a handful?
- » Asking for sauces to be served on the side so you can control how much you eat, as many sauces can be sugary, salty, creamy and made with poor-quality oils.
- » An entree-sized meal as a main, or main for an entree, whatever suits your needs best.
- » If certain foods upset your digestive system or you have an allergy, ask about ingredients. Some people need to minimise garlic and onions, for example. If you are eating out the night before an event and feeling nervous, choose a lighter, more quickly digested option (e.g. a Napoli pasta over carbonara, grilled fish over deep- or shallow-fried) – something you know works for you.
- » Feeling like dessert but a bit full already? Share one – that way you get the taste and the experience without the overfull feeling.
- » A restaurant should always be able to prepare grilled meat or fish with vegetables, even if it's not on the menu. Contact the restaurant prior to organise this.
- » If you need more carbohydrates, order extra bread or rolls, a side of steamed rice or a bowl of potatoes or sweet potatoes.

Remember, it's okay to leave something on your plate if you have had enough. When we've paid for food, we don't like to leave it, but feeling overfull is no fun, and is costly to health and performance. Remind yourself how horrible it feels when you can't sleep because you have eaten too much. Sleep is very important for health, preparation and recovery, so we want to avoid interfering with it. Listening to your appetite can be key to maximising the performance benefit you get from food, rather than hindering it.

EATING BREAKFAST OUT

It's become popular to go for a bike ride and then have breakfast at a cafe or something similar. If you do this regularly, choose where and what you eat wisely. Breakfast may be your recovery meal, so it is important. Aim to have some protein for muscle recovery, wholegrain carbohydrate to replace the energy used, and fruit or vegetables with some healthy fats for overall repair and health. Modify your order depending on what this meal is needed for. Following are some suggestions:

- The egg and bacon roll could instead be a wholegrain roll or wrap with some vegetables thrown in, or a cooked breakfast of eggs, mushrooms, tomato, spinach and avocado, with wholegrain toast and a rasher of bacon.
- Instead of sliced fruit toast and butter, try wholegrain fruit toast with ricotta and banana to boost the nutritional value.
- Smashed avocado on toast could have added protein such as feta, ricotta cheese, tasty cheese, baked beans, smoked salmon, an egg or tofu.
- Porridge and Bircher muesli are great choices, offering protein, carbohydrate and fluid. If needing to boost the kilojoule value of these, some skim milk or protein powder could be stirred in.
- Juices and smoothies are all the rage, but quench your thirst with water first. Be careful of large fruit juices. They contain 10 per cent sugar – you may or may not want this much carbohydrate. If you are struggling to keep weight up and need more kilojoules then juice might be an easy way to achieve this. If extra protein is needed, a milkshake with milk, yoghurt, fruit and a few chia seeds could be an option. Why not ask for your own combination of ingredients if they're not on the menu?

A vegetable-based juice will give an electrolyte boost from the potassium and the vitamins and minerals. A veggie juice can be a great way to boost your vegetable intake, remembering that minerals such as calcium and iron in vegetables are less well absorbed by the body than they are from animal sources. If you are relying on vegetables as your main sources of these minerals, such as in a vegan diet, it's important to have a variety of sources and to consume extra to allow for the poor absorption.

BUYING LUNCH

If you are buying lunch, think about including vegetables (these can often be lacking, even in a vegetarian meal), protein and carbohydrate. Follow the same principle as when you're making lunch yourself. Don't be scared to ask for additions and subtractions to foods – after all, you are the customer.

Some suggestions:

- Avoid overeating, as this can make you feel sluggish later. Buy less, or eat half at lunch and the other half later. Sometimes cafe-bought sandwiches can be enormous. Make sure you stop when you feel comfortable – you should be around 7/10–8/10 full.
- It's hard to know the quality of the oils and fats used when you're buying lunch, so skip areas where they are likely to be poor, such as deep-fried food and margarine on bread. Extra virgin olive oil is the way to go.
- If you're going out for a burger and you want to make it more nutritious, choose a wholegrain or wholemeal bun if possible. If you're getting full, leave some, for example the bun, and just eat the filling. Also, go for grilled meat or a fish fillet, and make sure you get plenty of salad.
- Have a risotto containing equal portions of rice, vegetables and meat, instead of a pile of rice.
- Try having salad and lean meat, egg or cheese on a sandwich or wrap.
- Choose grilled or oven-steamed fish (try Asian style), salad, wholegrain bread, legumes or steamed brown rice.
- Jacket potato can be a great option, with loads of filling choices such as lean mince, tuna, beans (legumes), salsa, mushrooms, corn, coleslaw (made with natural yoghurt dressing) and cheese.
- Mexican food offers a range of options – you can have burritos in a bowl with salad, beans or meat and brown rice, or the standard burrito if you need more carbohydrate for high energy.

SUSHI AND RICE PAPER ROLLS

Sushi and rice paper rolls are both popular lunch options. Sushi has a lot of rice compared to filling. The rice is short-grain and digested quickly, so if you are looking for quick energy, sushi will give you that. It's a great carbohydrate boost when needed, as a pre- or post-training snack, for in between sessions or for replenishing carbohydrate stores during a carnival event requiring a top up of energy.

However, it's important to be aware of this if lots of carbohydrate is not what you are looking for. One or two sushi rolls followed with a bowl of miso soup, or salad, to give you more vegetables, and some extra protein such as egg, tuna, salmon or a small can of beans, works well if you are looking for more balance. Sushi on its own is very carbohydrate-heavy – brown rice or quinoa are better options.

Rice paper rolls tend to have more balance between the vegetables, protein source and noodles in the filling, generally making them a healthier choice. Making your own rice paper rolls or sushi is a great option as this means you can add more protein and vegetables to the filling, and, in the case of sushi, make the rice layer thinner. My kids love making their own, and I have also shown footballers how easy it is to do this. It's much more economical, too.

FOOD HYGIENE WHEN EATING OUT

When eating out, a sandwich or wrap is generally an easy winner because you can choose ingredients to meet your needs. However, it can be a high-risk food choice food safety–wise, depending on the ingredients chosen. Look for clean venues making freshly made sandwiches, where you choose the ingredients and can see that they look fresh.

Sandwiches contain ingredients like salad and cold protein sources (e.g. meat and fish) that are often sitting in containers for some time and will not be cooked, meaning bacteria levels can rapidly increase. Observe the preparation area, refrigeration and overall hygiene before ordering.

ORDERING GROUP MEALS WHEN EATING OUT

If a group of athletes will be eating out together, it might be worthwhile contacting the venue prior to talk through modifications to the menu. Suitable options might include fresh fruit platters with dipping coulis or yoghurt for dessert, wholegrain bread rolls, large green salads or bowls of vegetables on the table, and hearty minestrone soup or similar for entrees. If some members of the group have large appetites, the venue might need to know to provide larger servings.

For a main meal the night before an AFL game, I have moved away from buffet-style meals as much as possible. It can be so easy to eat a bit of everything and end up with an overloaded plate and a feeling of exhaustion from overeating. Players need to fuel themselves for the game the following day, but should not go overboard. After all, they will have a chance to eat breakfast and a snack before the game, too.

If you are setting up a buffet, think about the order of food placement. If a carbohydrate focus is required, put these dishes first. If you are feeding a group of athletes that need to keep body weight down, have the salads and vegetables at the start to fill up on the lower-kilojoule, nutrient-dense foods, and place the protein and carbohydrates foods further along. If there is a mix of requirements, people can start serving the foods they wish to first, and won't necessarily follow the order of the buffet table, though this could get chaotic with a big group.

When I order lunch for groups of sporting teams I request a build-your-own sandwich bar. All the ingredients are laid out with a variety of breads and the players make their own. This works well pre-game, where some players want to eat heavier meals with salad and cheese or meats on wholegrain breads, and others like lighter options and might make a banana, plain cheese or nut spread sandwich on wholemeal bread.

When working with the Australian Men's Cricket team, for example, some fast bowlers were going to bowl straight after lunch, so a white or wholemeal bread toasted cheese sandwich might be more suitable, as it can be digested rapidly, whereas a fielder might look for more sustained energy and choose a wholegrain salad sandwich. This is quite individual.

If you are ordering food for your team at a venue, consider the variety needed depending on how the meal fits in with training or competition. Lunch after a morning training session might need to be quite large, and if it was an endurance training session, plenty of carbohydrate foods should be provided. If it was a strength session, there should be plenty of protein choices. Will there be another training session in the afternoon? If so, lunch needs to be easily digested – some liquid foods such as smoothies and soups for fluid and electrolytes can be good options.

CHAPTER 19
Eating at Celebrations

Celebrations are a constant for most of us, including birthdays, anniversaries, New Year, Christmas, religious festivals, weddings – the list goes on. Our health and performance goals would certainly suffer if we were to overeat and drink on all of these occasions. Enjoying festivities is important, but being able to choose the food you want to eat and say no to what you don't without having to explain yourself is key to the enjoyment. It's important that athletes, particularly younger athletes, have the confidence to remind others around them (such as well-meaning family members) of their goals. A gentle reminder is usually sufficient for people to understand and be supportive. Most people won't actually notice what you choose to eat and drink unless you bring their attention to it.

Once people find out I am a dietitian, they often comment on the food I eat at parties. It can be annoying and feel like people are judging what I eat: 'Are you allowed to eat that cake? You're a dietitian!' Athletes often encounter similar comments: 'Are you allowed to eat that?' or 'Is that part of your training diet?' On the other hand, athletes eating healthy choices often have the opposite thrown at them: 'Oh come on, one won't hurt, eat up!' Sticking to your own plan can be difficult, particularly in the face of peer pressure. Make your own decision and remember that the people making the comments often don't have the same goals as you. Stick to what you want – there's no right or wrong, and you should be able to make your choice without judgement from others.

I don't understand the predominance of low-nutritional-value food that's traditionally offered at parties and celebrations. Quality over quantity, I say. I would prefer a quality, freshly made sandwich over a sausage roll or chips any day.

SURVIVING THE CELEBRATION

Whether you have the job of hosting the celebration or are a guest, here are some tips to help keep you feeling energised.

1. **Mindset:** Firstly, start thinking about food that is nourishing for your health, vitality and training. It's your party, after all (or your platter that you are taking to the party). Serve food that will have your guests feeling energised and their tastebuds tantalised. They will be thankful that they don't have to navigate traditional party fare as the only option.

2. **Veggies first in planning:** Start planning the menu with vegetables first and work backwards to the meats. There is an extensive range of antipasto platters you can make (roasted capsicum, eggplant, artichokes, sundried tomatoes, olives and pickled vegetables), and salads that are much more than a bowl of lettuce and tomato wedges. Try salads with added seeds, nuts, an array of greens (spinach, kale, rocket, broccoli, green beans), red cabbage, a variety of carrots and tomatoes – the list goes on. Salad dressings don't have to be time consuming, either. A good extra virgin olive oil, vinegar and a sprinkle of herbs can do the trick.

   For other vegetable ideas, look at how much people love a traditional roast. Plan the vegetables as the big feature and then add meat in smaller amounts. Roasted sweet potato, pumpkin, potato, zucchini, capsicum, tomato, mushroom and beetroot are all great options. A barbecue can be planned in the same way, with more vegetables and salads and less of the meat.

   Vegetable curries and soups in winter and capsicum, snow peas and carrots with dips are all delicious ways to increase the vegetables on offer.

3. **Protein source:** Meat, as the traditional protein source, tends to be the focus when planning menus. Try seafood instead, it's often a winner, or legumes and lentils and soy-based protein (falafels, bean salads, Mexican beans, minestrone soup, tofu in stir-fry). A platter of prawns or fish on the barbecue are also delicious.

   If cooking meat, there is a range to choose from, including kangaroo, lean beef, lamb, pork, chicken and goat. Combine these with plant proteins such as legumes or lentils, which make great burgers and additions to salads. Skewers or kebabs mixed with meat and vegetables provide a good balance. Make your own souvlaki, encouraging plenty of salad. If people are serving themselves, have the meat at the end of the table so they start with vegetables and salads first.

Buying a lot of meat and seafood can be expensive, so think 'vegetables first', with smaller serves of meat and seafood. Some plant protein sources, such as tofu, can help balance the budget and provide valuable nutritious options as well.

4. **Your nutritional needs:** Cook or take a dish that is going to suit your nutritional needs. Make it work the best you can to meet your needs. For example:
    a. Is it the day before a game or race and you have a traditional favourite you would like to eat?
    b. Will the celebration be after a match or long training session, when you need protein and carbohydrate, and a bigger meal?
    c. Will you be going to training afterwards, and so need a lighter meal?

5. **Leftovers:** If you are the host and there are leftovers you don't want to eat, send them home with others. Make it easy for you to eat how you would like to.

6. **Dessert:** I do love a good dessert, but sometimes find that people go overboard with serving sizes. Cut cake into small serves for people to enjoy. Depending what is in season, go for bowls or plates of fresh fruit, berries, cherries, pineapple and watermelon. A cheese platter with grapes, nuts, fresh apricots and sliced pear can be just what people like to finish off the meal.

7. **Drinks:** Have plenty of non-alcoholic and non-sweetened beverages available. For those not drinking alcohol, a sugar-laden drink is not necessarily the preferred choice. Try these options instead:
    » jugs of water with slices of lemon, lime, mint leaves or sliced strawberries
    » soda water or natural mineral water

- » kombucha – this is a low-sugar, alcohol-free fermented tea drink that contains bacteria and yeast. I encourage the athletes I work with to use the commercially available varieties that have been fermented under Australian Food Standards manufacturing conditions. You can also make kombucha at home, but ensure you are brewing it correctly, as a nasty colony of bacteria can form. Kombucha has a cider-type taste, similar to an alcoholic drink, but without the alcohol or sugar. It is thought to have some gut health benefits too, though research is still being done in this area.
- » a special selection of tea and coffee.

Be aware of how much alcohol you are drinking, and space alcoholic drinks out with water and other alternatives.

KIDS' PARTY TIPS

There may be some periods in your life when children's parties are a frequent event. It can be fun to have some traditional 'party food', but it's a good idea to also provide some great-tasting, nutritious food for growing bodies. This isn't about depriving anyone, it's about making healthy choices easy options.

This is particularly important for very sporty children who are training and growing. Some have extra nutritional requirements for their sports, and offering nutritious food choices makes it easier for them to meet their needs. Adults often attend children's parties too, and when kids are young there can sometimes be several parties in the same week.

Here are some suggestions to consider:

- » **What to drink?** Yes, it is a party, but I would still encourage water as the main drink, possibly in fun jugs, cool cups, or kids' own bottles – they could even decorate their bottle with stickers or markers. When they were older, my children wanted soft drink, so we had some available, along with 100 per cent fruit juice, water and milk. Milkshakes with fruit, milk and yoghurt/ice cream can also be fun. For bigger kids, soda water or natural mineral water with fruit slices is a good option.

- » **What to eat?** What is your child's favourite food? It might be spaghetti or hamburgers, roast chicken or sushi. Base the party food around this, rather than the stereotypical food – it's their birthday, after all. When he was in primary school, my son loved spaghetti bolognaise, so we had bowls of it, along with homemade chicken nuggets, homemade meat pies (which did take far too long to make) and a standard birthday cake. The kids loved it. At one Sri Lankan child's birthday party I attended, traditional rice and curry was served and all the kids ate and enjoyed it. I came home with a bag of the spices to make it at home! Another easy and popular option is hamburgers or kebabs. They can be homemade, with salad fillings and wraps or bread rolls on a platter so kids can construct their own.

- » **Swap the chips:** Instead of chips, try some other options. Pikelets (either savoury or sweet), homemade popcorn, roasted chickpeas, dried fruit, toasted pita bread with extra virgin olive oil and sprinkled with herbs, pretzels and rice crackers and, if there are no allergies, nuts can be good for older kids. The main issue with chips is the poor-quality oil they are cooked in and the excessive amount of salt.

- » **Combine food and fun:** Having food that people can construct themselves allows everyone to modify for taste and nutritional needs. At my own children's parties over the years I've had:

    - » **Make your own pizza:** My children enjoyed make your own pizza parties in kindergarten. I gave each child a ball of homemade dough and had an array of ingredients available in the middle for them to make their own. Banging out the dough kept them amused for some time. (We did this outside to save cleaning up all the flour.) This can also be a winner when having a combination of adult and younger guests – everyone can make their own to suit.

    - » **Decorate and bake cupcakes:** This was a hit when my daughter was eleven. It involves lots of sugar (though you could do muffins with savoury ingredients or fruit), but it's still developing cooking skills, and it followed a barbecue of chicken breast, bread rolls and salad, so we still had a nourishing meal.

    - » **Make your own sushi and rice paper rolls:** When my daughter started high school, sushi was all the rage. The ingredients were laid out and the girls made their own. These can be nutritionally varied to meet your training needs, with extra vegetables or protein filling with less noodles, or more noodles if needed for recovery or carbohydrate loading before an endurance event.

Poke bowls are now popular – you can put an array of ingredients out and people can make their own. This gives them control of what they eat.

» **Hunt:** As a child I loved going to one particular girl's party every year. Her mum gave us a brown paper bag each and hid peanuts in their shells around the backyard. You had to find as many as you could to win. The peanuts were fresh, and shelling them was a novelty. It beats a lolly hunt for something different! (If nuts are a no-go, try hiding something else instead – apart from Easter eggs.)

NUTRITION TIPS FOR CHRISTMAS

It's beginning to look a lot like Christmas ... how will you survive? There can be so many end-of-year parties, family gatherings and celebrations to attend. If you don't keep an eye on what you eat and drink, instead of feeling refreshed after a break from work, you can end up starting the new year feeling sluggish.

Don't feel that you have to overindulge. This is not the last celebration – more will come. In fact, think about the good health you are gaining, and see this as part of your training, rather than approaching it with a mindset of missing out. You are nurturing yourself by making nutritional choices that suit you. Here are a few tips to make things easier on yourself and avoid compromising your training and performance while still enjoying yourself.

1. **Keep festive fare special:** Have whatever you like on Christmas Day. I leave the Christmas cake, mince pies and other celebratory foods in the shops until the week before. Keep them special, rather than eating them for months prior. I take the same approach to Easter – I refuse to buy hot cross buns in January, when Easter isn't until April. It takes the excitement of waiting out of it.

2. **Choose:** When there is a range of foods offered, choose which of these foods you most desire, take a serving, eat and enjoy. Pause before having more. There is nothing to say you have to try everything – sometimes less is more.

3. **Plan:** What social activities are coming up? When will I enjoy an alcoholic drink and when will I reach for the water? Without a plan, before we know it, we've had more alcohol than intended, and feel below-par before Christmas has even arrived. The same goes for food. If you know you have a few functions in one week, you can pace yourself. If you'll be eating out in the evening, be sure to include plenty of vegetables with lunch. Think about what you need to fuel your upcoming training.

   I don't drink alcohol, and people often question why I don't. (I don't ask them why they do.) It can become tiring when people push you to have a drink, but I have found that by saying 'no thanks' convincingly, they tend not to ask again. Sometimes others want you to join in without realising it's because they're trying to make themselves feel better about their own choices. Stick to your guns. It's your choice.

4. **Serve one plate:** Buffet-style eating can be dangerous. By the time you get to the end your plate is often piled high, flavours are all mixed and it becomes a culinary shambles. And if you eat it all, you will probably wind up lying on the couch moaning about having overeaten and feeling lethargic. This is not what you need when you are training. Go for quality over quantity, sit down, savour the flavours and consider stopping before the 'full gauge' hits 10. You are likely to feel much better afterwards, and will still have enjoyed the meal.

5. **Go for five vegetables:** Aim for five servings of vegetables per day – it's always good to aim high. As it is the festive season and you want to make it special, go the extra mile with preparation. Roast a variety of vegetables, carrots (try a range of different colours), stuffed peppers, mushrooms, sweet potato, pumpkin and parsnip along with the traditional potatoes, using herbs and good oils. Make salads with roasted beetroot, radishes, leafy greens and summer tomatoes that are fresh and in season. Serve vegetables onto your plate first so they are the feature.

6. **Berries and cherries:** These are beautiful at summertime. Base desserts, pre-dinner nibbles or snacks for guests around these special fruits. They will leave you feeling refreshed, rather than heavy. One Easter I had my extended family over and everyone brought a plate of afternoon tea to share. Cakes were abundant, but the most popular option was the bowl of plump, sweet cherries that my cousin had picked from a cherry farm that day.
7. **Hydration:** Keep well hydrated with water.
    » Put out jugs of water when friends come over.
    » Take a water bottle when out and about running last-minute errands.
    » Start with a water before drinking alcohol when out socialising, and finish the evening with more. A hangover is mostly dehydration. If you are going to be training the next day and plan on having a few more alcoholic beverages than usual, you may need to up the water and electrolyte-based drinks.
    » We can also confuse thirst with hunger, so start with some water.
8. **Sizes:** Look at the size of your plates, bowls and glasses. Keep these smaller, to help manage portion sizes. This is particularly important if you participate in a sport where you need to keep to a weight category. You want to enjoy the festive season without paying for it over the future months. Listen to your body's signals and needs, at least most of the time.
9. **Gifts:** Consider gifts that are not the traditional last-minute box of chocolates, and suggest that family and friends try to do the same. Each year I make a small hamper for each of the staff at the doctor's clinic where I consult. They look forward to the Christmas goodies, home-made fruit cake and biscuits, and I also add a bottle of nice oil, some fresh nuts or a Christmas ornament. It is always a winner, and provides a bit of balance.

GIFT SHOPPING

Limited time and money can make buying gifts tricky. Here are a few foodie options to ask for or purchase.

1. **Walking tours:** There's a huge range of walking tours available all over the world, including gourmet food, coffee, tea, market and dumpling tours. See what your city has to offer and buy a voucher.
2. **Vinegar:** A quality bottle of balsamic or other vinegar is always a winner. Check for local growers.
3. **Extra virgin olive oil:** Some good Australian extra virgin olive oil is the perfect companion gift for a nice vinegar. Look for the triangle indicating that the oil is approved extra virgin olive oil.
4. **Fruit:** A box of cherries, mangoes, grapes, peaches, berries or a combination of seasonal fruits is a special treat to be shared.
5. **Bamboo cutting boards:** These can even be ordered with personalised messages. I love the light–hard combination and the ease of cleaning and drying. Chopping boards should be changed regularly to ensure good hygiene – most of us don't do this often enough, so they are a perfect, useful gift.
6. **Herbs and spices:** Pots of fresh herbs ready for festive feasts and fresh summer salads can make a great gift. You can also find some interesting spice mixes, which can be a winner.
7. **Subscription:** A subscription to a magazine on health, sport, the outdoors or gourmet travel can be an ongoing monthly treat.
8. **Tea towels:** Practical and boring to some, I always appreciate a quality tea towel that dries well. Use it as the wrapping paper for the next suggestion.

9. **Chutneys, sauces, mustards or preserves:** Homemade varieties make particularly nice gifts – I always appreciate the love and time that has gone into making them, and their superior taste. Fermented vegetables are all the rage for gut health, too – have a go. Get together with some friends to make a batch before Christmas.
10. **Containers:** Ornamental glass jars or sturdy plastic containers can be filled with layers of nuts, seeds, dried fruit, homemade preserves or ingredients that can be combined to make a muesli, cake or spices for a meal. For a busy athlete, that would be a dream. Attach the recipe so they can refill and reuse the container for a new batch.

Edible, healthy gifts don't collect dust and can be shared with family and friends.

CHAPTER 20
Healthy Eating While Travelling

Do you travel regularly for work, for leisure or for your sport? Elite athletes are often travelling – I have organised many an interstate or overseas meal. For me, no matter where I am, the focus is always on enjoying food and eating, particularly when there are new local foods and cuisines to explore.

HAVE A SNACK ON HAND

When travelling it can be a good habit to have a snack on hand, in case flights, trains, buses or traffic jams will delay you. For elite athletes, keeping to a schedule of eating and drinking is important, both physically and psychologically. You don't want to be playing catch-up late at night due to poor access to food during the day.

Recently I attended a professional development event where I caught up with a dietitian I had studied with twenty years ago. We were sitting together and I said I was getting hungry, to which she replied, 'You know what I always remember about you? You always had a snack with you when we were at uni!' I was surprised – I didn't think this was noteworthy. I like to be prepared, and always make sure I have some fuel on hand. People are not at their best when hungry and tired from travelling. Dynamics are important for any travelling team, whether it's a sporting team, travelling buddies or work colleagues, so making sure people are adequately fuelled has many benefits.

STRATEGIES FOR SUCCESS WHILE TRAVELLING

There's a common misconception that when you are on holidays, you need to overeat to enjoy yourself, and this tends to involve lots of low-nutritional-value foods. If I do this, I find that the holiday is much less enjoyable, as I feel sluggish and heavy, and my bowels get out of kilter. I do enjoy indulging, but I make sure I only do it to a point where I still feel well.

If you're travelling for work, the challenge may be that healthy choices are limited by time and availability. It's also easy to forget that the travel isn't a holiday! Travelling frequently for work without having healthy eating strategies in place can really affect your health and performance.

Here are some tips for positive health and performance outcomes while on your travels.

FRESH FRUIT AND VEGETABLES

Due to customs and quarantine laws (unless you're travelling within your state), you are unlikely to be able to take fresh fruit or vegetables with you, so you'll need to buy locally when you arrive. If you're travelling locally, a loaded-up cooler bag or Esky works well – apples, oranges, mandarins, carrots, lettuce, tomatoes and cucumber all travel fairly well.

If you're travelling on business, particularly if you stay in the same accommodation regularly, you could:

» Order a fruit basket to be waiting in your room.
» Do a supermarket shop online and arrange for the groceries to be delivered to your accommodation. Include breakfast, lunch and snack items to keep you healthy and energised, and to save time and money.

BREADS

Wraps, mountain bread or wholegrain dry biscuits with a nut spread, Vegemite, canned fish or baked beans are all non-perishable and can travel. Local cheeses with tomato can be added at any time for breakfast, lunch or a snack. I have been known to buy smoked salmon, local cheese and a few salad items to chop up for a platter by the pool while on holidays. It's nourishing and delicious, and prevents us from ordering takeaway or eating the mini bar.

NUTS, DRIED FRUIT, TRAIL MIX

These are great options when driving or waiting for planes, trains or other transport. If you're hiking or doing lots of walking, they're great for restoring energy. I remember nibbling a few while driving from Cairns to Cape Tribulation.

BREAKFAST CEREAL

Bringing your own breakfast, such as cereal (with some camping bowls and spoons) to your accommodation works well. It's easy to overeat by going out or eating at the hotel buffet, causing you to feel sluggish. I love to get up and look out at the local scenery while eating breakfast from or near my room before heading out to enjoy the day. Milk is usually supplied, but if not, some small packets of long-life milk will travel well. Cereal helps keep your fibre intake up to keep those bowels working, and it's easy and convenient.

MUESLI BARS

Bars are non-perishable and can even be eaten if they've been squashed at the bottom of a bag. They can be lifesavers if you're delayed at an airport, when the kids are hungry in the car, when you're out sightseeing, or between meetings. Choose the more nourishing bars containing nuts, oats, seeds, fruit and less added sugars.

EQUIPMENT

Pack some cutlery, bowls and plates – even a toasted sandwich maker can be a hit (especially if you're travelling with kids). You can whip up a baked bean, cheese or tuna toastie. It won't take up as much room in your suitcase as you think.

You can also take a kettle. In some parts of Europe these aren't supplied in standard accommodation. Couscous or rice vermicelli noodles just need hot water added. Stir through some flavoured canned fish or beans and, if you're lucky enough to have some available, a handful of spinach. It might not be the most balanced meal, but it's better than raiding the mini bar when you're tired, it's late or the budget has become tight.

When the kids were young I took the electric frying pan along on a holiday to use on nights they were too tired to venture out for dinner. We had a great time travelling with a friend, who is also a dietitian, and her kids. The electric frying pan made cooking feel like indoor camping. It was great fun, and you'd be amazed at what you can cook! We cooked homemade hamburgers, local fresh fish and oven chips (our oven was the pan with the lid on), and pancakes and eggs for breakfast. I'm not sure who had more fun – the adults, seeing what we could cook up in limited conditions, or the kids, watching us cook in the bathroom with the fan on to make sure we didn't set off the smoke alarms in the apartment.

Cricketer Matthew Hayden, who is a keen cook, used to pack a bread maker and rice cooker on long tours to India. He would also visit chefs in the hotel kitchen and learn about local cooking.

I have worked with swimmers who take rice cookers on trips to use in hotel rooms – you just need to plug them in, and you can throw in vegetables and meat along with the rice. This gives the athletes much more control over what they are eating, and it won't set off any smoke alarms like a toaster might.

BOOKING ACCOMMODATION

When you're booking accommodation, remember that having food preparation facilities will make life much easier. I like a small kitchenette, or at least a bar fridge. That way I can make breakfast with freshly bought local fruit, yoghurt and cereal (sometimes from home). Before booking, find out if there's a local supermarket or store nearby to pick up basics.

If you are going to be out and about all day, and especially if you're venturing to places where food won't be available for purchase, such as on bush walks, taking food is essential. This can be more than a Vegemite sandwich (even though they're pretty good, especially with avocado). When walking at Mossman Gorge I pack gourmet style: smoked salmon, local cheeses and sourdough breads, macadamia nuts and fresh mango with some cold packs, and a little chocolate for dessert.

I was travelling with the Australian Men's Cricket team in Hobart once, and the players had a day off so a couple went fishing, hoping to catch something we could all eat that night. Ricky Ponting wasn't convinced that Andrew Symonds and crew would catch enough, so I accompanied Matthew Hayden and Ricky Ponting down to Hobart's dock, where they bought some local seafood. Andrew Symonds did catch some fish that day, but it was lucky we'd also bought some. Matthew Hayden and Andrew Symonds cooked up a storm in the small apartment they were staying in, and we all ate a feast of seafood. Being away sometimes means you have more time to cook than you would at home, so make the most of the opportunity.

BOOKING FLIGHTS

When booking flights, you can request special meals in advance, if desired. This is especially important if you have an allergy or intolerance, as you don't want to skip meals for long periods. Being too hungry makes life unpleasant, reduces your energy levels and can impair performance. You may need to take extra food with you, as plane meals can be small, and you are stuck if you don't like it. I have hit a roadblock in the past when requesting extra food for players, being told that it won't fit on the tray. My solution has been to order food for athletes to eat prior to boarding, such as meat and salad rolls, and for breakfast flights, packs made up and delivered with Bircher muesli or quiche slices, fruit and nut slices, yoghurt and fruit salad. You could contact a venue at an airport to have them ready for you to pick up, and eat them while waiting in the lounge.

CLUB LOUNGES

If you have airline club lounge access there can be some good choices available. Food is usually buffet-style, so try to stick to your usual routine and don't get carried away. Soup will help with maintaining hydration due to the fluid and sodium. Limit or avoid alcohol, as it's dehydrating, and a plane flight is dehydrating enough. Stick to the sparkling water, or have a cup of tea.

EATING LOCAL/EATING OUT

It is lovely to visit local restaurants – trying new foods is part of what travelling is about. When visiting the Daintree Rainforest in Queensland the local bananas were a highlight, and they made a convenient and portable energy boost. When in Asia, the local fruits such as mangoes and pineapples are divine. In Vietnam, my kids love buying fresh pineapple at the market – they cut it up for you in ready-to-eat quarters. When we visited Italy some years ago, our afternoon snack was gelati and raspberries, which kept us going between a light lunch and the evening meal.

It's okay to ask for modifications to the menu – extra salad or vegetables, and no or less chips. If you would like to try a few different items, share with others, or order two entrees instead of an entree and a main, and share dessert. These points are particularly relevant if you're travelling frequently, or for a few weeks at once. If you travel a few days every month this adds up to a month or more a year, so it's worth thinking about the nutrition of the meals. That's a decent amount of your food intake, and therefore your health and performance.

Do you take road trips for work or to reach your training or competition venue? If you're not packing your meals, try pre-planning where you are going to stop en route, as roadside service stations and fast-food outlets will have limited suitable choices. If organising team meals on a road trip, I suggest calling a local restaurant to see what they can provide. If the menu they offer doesn't quite suit, discuss options. Confirm by calling ahead to let them know how far away your bus is – this means the food will be ready not long after arrival, keeping you on schedule, and it also ensures they haven't forgotten. Planning means you are less likely to deviate and go to the closest drive-through because you are tired and can't be bothered looking elsewhere. Make the healthy choices the easy choices.

If a competition is soon, I encourage foods that offer minimal risk of food poisoning, particularly in countries where hygiene standards are lower than what you are used to. Seafood and raw foods including salad are higher-risk options. Ensure that hot food is very hot (above 60° Celsius) – I have had teams travelling overseas take thermometers to check temperatures of food – and make sure it hasn't been sitting around in a warmer for hours. If it is looking shrivelled, that is a clear sign that you should skip it.

FLUID

The time between leaving home and boarding a flight can involve several hours with minimal food and fluid. Keep drinking (not at the airport bar) to stay well hydrated before boarding – you don't want to start the flight partially dehydrated, particularly as the air in an aircraft cabin is dry, causing you to lose extra fluid through respiration. On long trips, either driving or flying, we sometimes reduce our fluid intake to avoid having to go to the toilet. This can leave you dehydrated, so try to keep the fluids up. It's worth having a cup or two of an oral rehydration fluid on a flight. Have a peek in the toilet bowl – your urine colour will tell you if you need to drink more. If it's dark and smelly, you need to dial up the water.

Conclusion

Eating like an athlete is about fuelling yourself optimally for any activity life presents. It can be a way of eating at any age, and is about being in tune with your body and enjoying your food for good health. Finding the right dietary intake for you is a bit like putting a jigsaw together, one piece at a time – you just need to move the pieces around until they create the right picture.

Notes